Anatomy and Physiology
of
Animals

Latest version at: http://en.wikibooks.org/wiki/Anatomy_and_Physiology_of_Animals

J. Ruth Lawson

This printed paperback edition published by Platypus Global Media (registered with US ISBN agency)

ISBN-13: 978-0615540337

Contents

Articles

References

Article Licenses

Anatomy and Physiology of Animals

Veterinary nurses need to have a firm grasp of the normal structure of an animal's body and how it functions before they can understand the effect diseases and injuries have and the best ways to treat them.

This book describes the structure of the animal body and the way in which it works. Animals encountered in normal veterinary practice are used as examples where possible. The material is divided into 16 chapters:

- Chemicals
- Classification
- The Cell
- Body Organisation
- The Skin
- The Skeleton
- Muscles
- Cardiovascular System
- Respiratory System
- Lymphatic System
- The Gut and Digestion
- Urinary System
- Reproductive System
- Nervous System
- The Senses
- Endocrine System

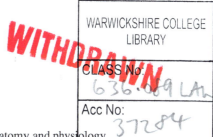

original image by tanakawho [1] cc by

Extra resources

- A Glossary gives the meaning of technical terms used in the text.
- There is a "Test Yourself" [2] for each chapter.
- Worksheets [3] are available on WikiEducator.
- WikiVet [4] - a free wiki for veterinary students with a detailed section on anatomy and physiology
- Presentations [5] of the material can be accessed by students of Otago Polytechnic who must use their polytechnic login to gain access.

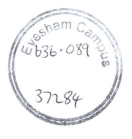

About the book

- Preface
- The Author
- Acknowledgements
- Table of contents

References

[1] http://flickr.com/photos/28481088@N00/290148609/

[2] http://www.wikieducator.org/The_Anatomy_and_Physiology_of_Animals/Test_Yourselves

[3] http://www.wikieducator.org/The_Anatomy_and_Physiology_of_Animals

[4] http://www.wikivet.net/

[5] http://blackboard.tekotago.ac.nz/webapps/portal/frameset.jsp?tab=courses&url=/bin/common/course.pl?course_id=_519_1&
bsession=311094&bsession_str=session_id%3D311094,user_id_pk1%3D,user_id_sos_id_pk2%3D,one_time_token%3D&
bsession_md5=c32686303e7a3a2446b0b013b7a9115d

Anatomy and Physiology of Animals/Preface

Preface by Ruth Lawson

This WikiBook "The Anatomy and Physiology of Animals' is designed to meet the needs of students studying for New Zealand certificate level qualifications in Veterinary Nursing, Animal Care and Rural Animal Technology under the New Zealand Qualifications Unit Standard 5180 [1]. It may also be useful for anyone studying for preliminary qualifications in veterinary nursing or biology. It is intended for use by students with little previous biological knowledge.

The WikiBook has been divided into 16 chapters covering fundamental concepts like organic chemistry, body organisation and the cell and then the systems of the body. Within each chapter are lists of Websites that provide additional information including animations. There is a comprehensive Glossary which can be accessed through links in each chapter. To help the student understand and learn the information within each chapter there are links to Worksheets in WikiEducator and a "Test Yourself" exercise.

The present text has evolved over many years. Terry Marler BVSC first conceived it as 8 separate modules for students at the Otago Polytechnic in what was then known as Animal Technology. Since then he and I have given it several major and minor overhauls. The present incarnation for this WikiBook has been rewritten and the diagrams redrawn by myself with advice and proofreading by Terry.

References

[1] http://www.nzqa.govt.nz/nqfdocs/units/pdf/5180.pdf

Anatomy and Physiology of Animals/The Author

Ruth Lawson is a zoologist who gained her first degree at Imperial College, London University and her D.Phil from York University, UK. After post graduate research on the tropical parasitic worm that causes schistosomiasis, she emigrated to New Zealand where she spent 10 years studying how hydatid disease spreads and can be controlled. With the birth of her daughter, Kate, she started to teach at the Otago Polytechnic, in Dunedin. Although human and animal anatomy and physiology has been her main teaching focus, she retains a strong interest and teaches courses in parasitology, public health, animal nutrition and pig husbandry. Ruth lives on the Otago Peninsula overlooking the beautiful Otago Harbour where she races her Topper sailing dinghy. She also enjoys tramping, skiing and gardening and has meditated for many years.

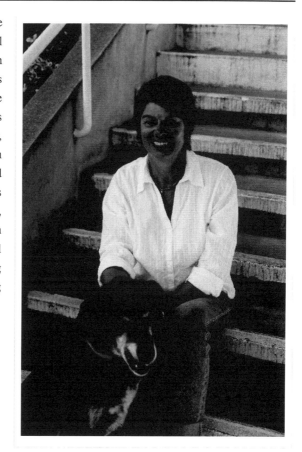

Anatomy and Physiology of Animals/Acknowledgements

Many thanks to Terry Marler (B.V.S.C.) for his guiding vision, wisdom, experience and patience. His advice throughout the writing of this WikiBook has been invaluable. I would also like to thank Bronwyn Hegarty, for gently shepherding the project through the many hurdles encountered and Leigh Blackall, also in the Education Development Unit at the Otago Polytechnic, for helpful discussions and advice. Many, many thanks also to Sunshine Blackall for her skills in formatting the diagrams and designing the artwork accompanying each chapter. The high quality of this work would not have been possible without the financial assistance of the Otago Polytechnic CAPEX fund. Thanks are also due to Jeanette O'Fee, my Head of School, for encouragement throughout the project and to Keith Allnatt and Jan Bedford for proofreading and reviewing. Finally I would like thank Peter and Kate who have patiently suffered my "unavailability" as I tapped my evenings and weekends away on the computer. *Ruth Lawson*

Anatomy and Physiology of Animals/Table of contents

Table of Contents for Print Version

Chapter 1 Chemicals

Chapter 2 Classification

Chapter 3 The Cell

Chapter 4 Body Organisation

Chapter 5 The Skin

Chapter 6 The Skeleton

Chapter 7 Muscles

Chapter 8 Cardiovascular System

Chapter 9 Respiratory System

Chapter 10 Lymphatic System

Chapter 11 The Gut and Digestion

Chapter 12 Urinary system

Chapter 13 Reproductive System

Chapter 14 Nervous System

Chapter 15 The Senses

Chapter 16 Endocrine System

Homeostasis and Feedback Control

Anatomy and Physiology of Animals/Chemicals

Objectives

After completing this section, you should know the:

- symbols used to represent atoms;
- names of molecules commonly found in animal cells;
- characteristics of ions and electrolytes;
- basic structure of carbohydrates with examples;
- carbohydrates can be divided into mono- di- and poly-saccharides;
- basic structure of fats or lipids with examples;
- basic structure of proteins with examples;
- function of carbohydrates, lipids and proteins in the cell and animals' bodies;
- foods which supply carbohydrates, lipids and proteins in animal diets.

Elements And Atoms

The elements (simplest chemical substances) found in an animal's body are all made of basic building blocks or atoms. The most common elements found in cells are given in the table below with the symbol that is used to represent them.

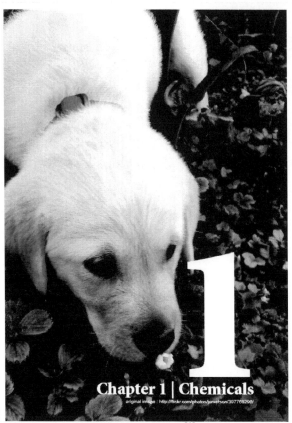

Chapter 1 | Chemicals
original image : http://flickr.com/photos/jurvetson/397768200/

original image by jurvetson [1] cc by

Atom	Symbol
Calcium	Ca
Carbon	C
Chlorine	Cl
Copper	Cu
Iodine	I
Hydrogen	H
Iron	Fe
Magnesium	Mg
Nitrogen	N
Oxygen	O
Phosphorous	P
Potassium	K
Sodium	Na
Sulfur	S

Zinc	Zn

Compounds And Molecules

A **compound** or **molecule** is formed when two or more **atoms** join together. Note that some atoms are never found alone. For example **oxygen** is always found as molecules of 2 oxygen atoms (represented as O_2).

The table below gives some common compounds.

Compound	Symbol
Calcium carbonate	$CaCO_3$
Carbon dioxide	CO_2
Copper sulfate	$CuSO_4$
Glucose	$C_6H_{12}O_6$
Hydrochloric acid	HCl
Sodium bicarbonate (baking soda)	$NaHCO_3$
Sodium chloride (table salt)	$NaCl$
Sodium hydroxide	$NaOH$
Water	H_2O

Chemical Reactions

Reactions occur when atoms combine with or separate from other atoms. In the process new products with different chemical properties are formed.

Chemical reactions can be represented by **chemical equations**. The starting atoms or compounds are usually put on the left-hand side of the equation and the products on the right-hand side.

For example

- $H_2O + CO_2$ gives H_2CO_3
- Water + Carbon dioxide gives Carbonic acid

Ionisation

When some atoms dissolve in water they become charged particles called **ions**. Some become positively charged ions and others negatively charged. Ions may have one, two or sometimes three charges.

The table below shows examples of positively and negatively charged ions with the number of their charges.

Positive Ions		Negative Ions	
H+	Hydrogen	Cl-	Chloride
Ca^{2+}	Calcium	OH-	Hydroxyl
Na+	Sodium	HCO_3^-	Bicarbonate
K+	Potassium	CO_3^{2-}	Carbonate
Mg^{2+}	Magnesium	SO_4^{2-}	Sulfate
Fe^{2+}	Iron (ferrous)	PO_4^{3-}	Phosphate
Fe^{3+}	Iron (ferric)	S^{2-}	Sulfide

Positive and negative ions attract one another to hold compounds together.

Ions are important in cells because they conduct electricity when dissolved in water. Substances that ionise in this way are known as **electrolytes**.

The molecules in an animal's body fall into two groups: **inorganic compounds** and **organic compounds**. The difference between these is that the first type does not contain **carbon** and the second type does.

Organic And Inorganic Compounds

Inorganic compounds include water, sodium chloride, potassium hydroxide and calcium phosphate.

Water is the most abundant inorganic compound, making up over 60% of the volume of cells and over 90% of body fluids like blood. Many substances dissolve in water and all the chemical reactions that take place in the body do so when dissolved in water. Other inorganic molecules help keep the **acid/base balance (pH)** and concentration of the blood and other body fluids stable (see Chapter 8).

Organic compounds include **carbohydrates, proteins** and **fats**. All organic molecules contain carbon atoms and they tend to be larger and more complex molecules than inorganic ones. This is largely because each carbon atom can link with four other atoms. Organic compounds can therefore consist of from one to many thousands of carbon atoms joined to form chains, branched chains and rings (see diagram below). All organic compounds also contain hydrogen and they may also contain other elements.

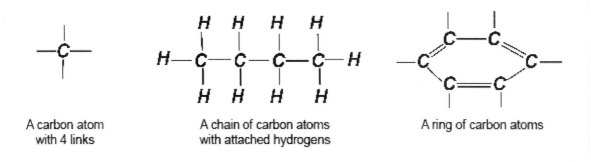

A carbon atom with 4 links   A chain of carbon atoms with attached hydrogens   A ring of carbon atoms

Carbohydrates

The name "carbohydrate" tells you something about the composition of these "hydrated carbon" compounds. They contain carbon, hydrogen and oxygen and like water (H_2O), there are always twice as many hydrogen atoms as oxygen atoms in each molecule. Carbohydrates are a large and diverse group that includes sugars, starches, glycogen and cellulose. Carbohydrates in the diet, supply an animal with much of its energy and in the animal's body, they transport and store energy.

Carbohydrates are divided into three major groups based on size: **monosaccharides** (single sugars), **disaccharides** (double sugars) and **polysaccharides** (multi sugars).

Monosaccharides are the smallest carbohydrate molecules. The most important monosaccharide is glucose which supplies much of the energy in the cell. It consists of a ring of 6 carbon atoms with oxygen and hydrogen atoms attached.

Disaccharides are formed when 2 monosaccharides join together. Sucrose (table sugar), maltose, and lactose (milk sugar), are three important disaccharides. They are broken down to monosaccharides by digestive enzymes in the gut.

Polysaccharides like starch, glycogen and cellulose are formed by tens or hundreds of monosaccharides linking together. Unlike mono- and di-saccharides, polysaccharides are not sweet to taste and most do not dissolve in water.

Glucose

Disaccharide (Lactose)

- **Starch** is the main molecule in which plants store the energy gained from the sun. It is found in grains like barley and roots like potatoes.
- **Glycogen**, the polysaccharide used by animals to store energy, is found in the liver and the muscles that move the skeleton.
- **Cellulose** forms the rigid cell walls of plants. Its structure is similar to glycogen, but it can't be digested by mammals. Cows and horses can eat cellulose with the help of bacteria which live in specialised parts of their gut.

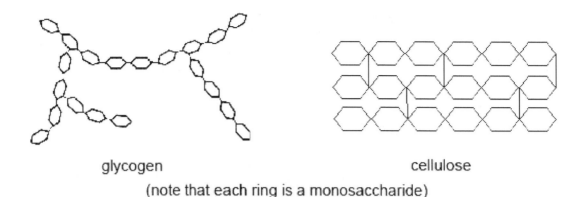

glycogen   cellulose

(note that each ring is a monosaccharide)

Fats

Fats or **lipids** are important in the plasma membrane around cells and form the insulating fat layer under the skin. They are also a highly concentrated source of energy, and when eaten in the diet provide twice as much energy per gram as either carbohydrates or proteins.

Like carbohydrates fats contain carbon, hydrogen and oxygen, but unlike them, there is no particular relationship between the number of hydrogen and oxygen atoms.

The fats and oils animals eat in their diets are called **triglycerides** or **neutral fats**. The building blocks of triglycerides are 3 **fatty acids** attached to a backbone of **glycerol (glycerine)**. When fats are eaten the digestive enzymes break down the molecules into separate fatty acids and glycerol again.

Fatty acids are divided into two kinds: **saturated** and **unsaturated fatty acids** depending on how much hydrogen they contain. The fat found in animals bodies and in dairy products contains mainly saturated fatty acids and tends to be solid at room temperature. Fish and poultry fats and plant oils contain mostly unsaturated fatty acids and are more liquid at room temperature.

Phospholipids are lipids that contain a phosphate group. They are important in the plasma membrane of the cell.

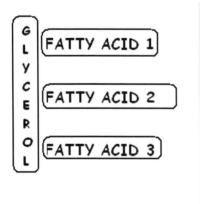

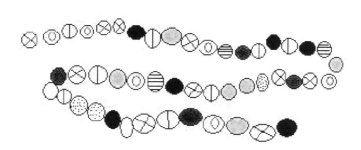

A chain of amino acids

Proteins

Proteins are the third main group of organic compounds in the cell - in fact if you dried out a cell you would find that about 2/3 of the dry dust you were left with would consist of protein. Like carbohydrates and fats, proteins contain C, H and O but they all also contain **nitrogen**. Many also contain sulphur and phosphorus.

In the cell, proteins are an important part of the plasma membrane of the cell, but their most essential role is as **enzymes**. These are molecules that act as biological catalysts and are necessary for biochemical reactions to proceed. Protein is also found as **keratin** in the skin, feathers and hair, in muscles, as well as in antibodies and some hormones.

Proteins are built up of long chains of smaller molecules called **amino acids**. There are 20 common types of amino acid and different numbers of these arranged in different orders create the multitude of individual proteins that exist in an animal's body.

Long chains of amino acids often link with other amino acid chains and the resulting protein molecule may twist, spiral and fold up to make a complex 3-dimensional shape. As an example, see the diagram of the protein lysozyme below. Believe it or not, this is a small and relatively simple protein.

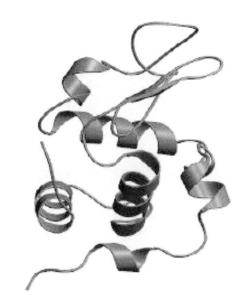

The protein lysozyme

It is this shape that determines how proteins behave in cells, particularly when they are acting as enzymes. If for any reason this shape is altered, the protein stops working. This is what happens if proteins are heated or put in a solution that is too acidic or alkaline. Think what happens to the "white'" of an egg when it is cooked. The "white" contains the protein albumin, which is changed or "**denatured**" permanently by cooking. The catastrophic effect that heat has on enzymes is one of the reasons animals die if exposed to high temperatures.

In the animal's diet, proteins are found in meat (muscle), dairy products, seeds, nuts and legumes like soya. When the enzymes in the gut digest proteins they break them down into the separate amino acids, which are small enough to be absorbed into the blood.

Summary

- **Ions** are charged particles, and **electrolytes** are solutions of ions in water.
- **Carbohydrates** are made of carbon with hydrogen and oxygen (in the same ratio as water) linked together. The cell mainly uses carbohydrates for energy.
- **Fats** are also made of carbon, hydrogen and oxygen. They are a powerful energy source, and are also used for insulation.
- **Proteins** are the building materials of the body, and as **enzymes** make cell reactions happen. They contain nitrogen as well as carbon, hydrogen and oxygen.

Worksheet

Worksheet on Chemicals in the Cell [2]

Test Yourself

1. What is the difference between an atom and a molecule?

2. What is the chemical name for baking soda?

> And its formula?

3. Write the equation for carbonic acid splitting into water and carbon dioxide.

4. A solution of table salt in water is an example of an electrolyte.

> What ions are present in this solution?

5. What element is always present in proteins but not usually in fats or carbohydrates?

6. List three differences between glucose and glycogen.

> 1.
>
> 2.
>
> 3.

7. Which will provide you with the most energy – one gram of sugar or one gram of butter?

Test Yourself Answers

Website

- Survey of the living world organic molecules [3]

A good summary of carbohydrates, fats and proteins.

Glossary

- Link to Glossary [4]

References

[1] http://flickr.com/photos/jurvetson/397768296/
[2] http://www.wikieducator.org/Chemicals_Worksheet
[3] http://darwin.baruch.cuny.edu/bio1003/organic_background.html
[4] http://en.wikibooks.org/wiki/Anatomy_and_Physiology_of_Animals/Glossary

Anatomy and Physiology of Animals/Chemicals/Test Yourself Answers

1. What is the difference between an atom and a molecule?

   An atom is the simplest building block of matter – elements are made of atoms. Molecules are made of atoms joined together.

2. What is the chemical name for baking soda? And its formula?

   Sodium Bicarbonate, NaHCO3

3. Write the equation for carbonic acid splitting into water and carbon dioxide.

H2CO3 • CO2 + H2O 4. A solution of table salt in water is an example of an electrolyte. What ions are present in this solution?

   Na+ and Cl- (also H+ and OH-)

5. What element is always present in proteins but not usually in fats or carbohydrates?

   Nitrogen

6. List three differences between glucose and glycogen.

   Glucose is a monosaccharide, glycogen is a polysaccharide (and a much bigger molecule); glucose is sweet to taste and dissolves in water, glycogen is not sweet and is insoluble; glucose is used for energy whereas glycogen stores energy.

7. Which will provide you with the most energy – one gram of sugar or one gram of butter?

   Fats provide approximately 2.5 times more energy than carbohydrates – so the butter wins hands down!

Anatomy and Physiology of Animals/Classification

Objectives

After completing this section, you should know:

- how to write the scientific name of animals correctly
- know that animals belong to the Animal kingdom and that this is divided into phyla, classes, orders, families
- know the definition of a species
- know the phylum and class of the more common animals dealt with in this course

Classification is the process used by scientists to make sense of the 1.5 million or so different kinds of living organisms on the planet. It does this by describing, naming and placing them in different groups. As veterinary nurses you are mainly concerned with the Animal Kingdom but don't forget that animals rely on the Plant Kingdom for food to survive. Also many diseases that animals are affected by are members of the other Kingdoms -- fungi, bacteria and single celled animals.

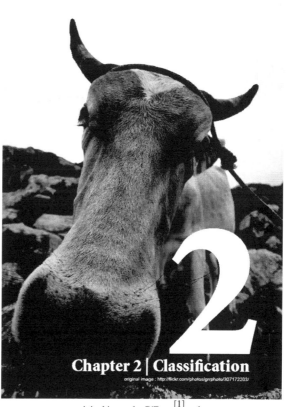

Chapter 2 | Classification
original image : http://flickr.com/photos/grrphoto/307172203/

original image by R'Eyes [1] cc by

Naming And Classifying Animals

There are more than 1.5 million different kinds of living organism on Earth ranging from small and simple bacteria to large, complex mammals. From the earliest time that humans have studied the natural world they have named these living organisms and placed them in different groups on the basis of their similarities and differences.

Naming Animals

Of course we know what a cat, a dog and a whale are but, in some situations using the common names for animals can be confusing. Problems arise because people in different countries, and even sometimes in the same country, have different common names for the same animals. For example a cat can be a chat, a Katze, gato, katt, or a moggie, depending on which language you use. To add to the confusion sometimes the same name is used for different animals. For example, the name 'gopher' is used for ground squirrels, rodents (pocket gophers), for moles and in the south-eastern United States for a turtle. This is the reason why all animals have been given an official **scientific** or **binomial name**. Unfortunately these names are always in Latin. For example:

- Common rat: *Rattus rattus*
- Human: *Homo sapiens*
- Domestic cat: *Felis domesticus*
- Domestic dog: *Canis familiaris*

As you can see from the above there are certain rules about writing scientific names:

- They always have **2 parts** to them.
- The first part is the **genus** name and is always written with a **capital** first letter.
- The second name is the **species** name and is always written in **lower case**.
- The name is always **underlined** or printed in **italics**.

The first time you refer to an organism you should write the whole name in full. If you need to keep referring to the same organism you can then abbreviate the genus name to just the initial. Thus "*Canis familiaris*" becomes "*C. familiaris*" the second and subsequent times you refer to it.

Classification Of Living Organisms

To make some sense of the multitude of living organisms they have been placed in different groups. The method that has been agreed by biologists for doing this is called the **classification system**. The system is based on the assumption that the process of evolution has, over the millennia, brought about slow changes that have converted simple one-celled organisms to complex multi-celled ones and generated the earth's incredible diversity of life forms. The classification system attempts to reflect the evolutionary relationships between organisms.

Initially this classification was based only on the appearance of the organism. However, the development of new techniques has advanced our scientific knowledge. The light microscope and later the electron microscope have enabled us to view the smallest structures, and now techniques for comparing DNA have begun to clarify still further the relationships between organisms. In the light of the advances in knowledge the classification has undergone numerous revisions over time.

At present most biologists divide the living world into 5 kingdoms, namely:

- bacteria
- protists
- fungi
- plants and
- animals

We are concerned here almost entirely with the **Animal Kingdom**. However, we must not forget that bacteria, protists, and fungi cause many of the serious diseases that affect animals, and all animals rely either directly or indirectly on the plant world for their nourishment.

The Animal Kingdom

So what are animals? If we were suddenly confronted with an animal we had never seen in our lives before, how would we know it was not a plant or even a fungus? We all intuitively know part of the answer to this.

Animals:

- eat organic material (plants or other animals)
- move to find food
- take the food into their bodies and then digest it
- and most reproduce by fertilizing eggs by sperm

If you were tempted to add that animals are furry, run around on four legs and give birth to young that they feed on milk you were thinking only of mammals and forgetting temporarily that frogs, snakes and crocodiles, birds as well as fish, are also animals.

These are all members of the group called the **vertebrates** (or animals with a backbone) and mammals make up only about 8% of this group. The diagram on the next page shows the percentage of the different kinds of vertebrates.

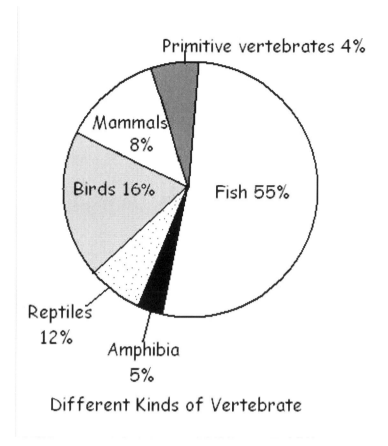

Different Kinds of Vertebrate

However, the term animal includes much more than just the Vertebrates. In fact this group makes up only a very small portion of all animals. Take a look at the diagram below, which shows the size of the different groups of animals in the Animal Kingdom as proportions of the total number of different animal species. Notice the small size of the segment representing vertebrates! All the other animals in the Animal Kingdom are animals with no backbone, or **invertebrates**. This includes the worms, sea anemones, starfish, snails, crabs, spiders and insects. As more than 90% of the invertebrates are insects, no wonder people worry that insects may take over the world one day!

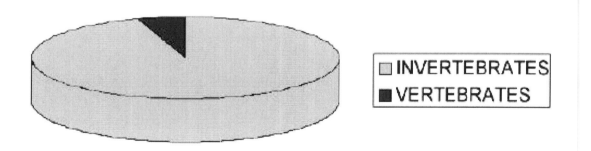

□ INVERTEBRATES
■ VERTEBRATES

The Classification Of Vertebrates

As we have seen above the Vertebrates are divided into 5 groups or classes namely:

- Fish
- Amphibia (frogs and toads)
- Reptiles (snakes and crocodiles)
- Birds
- Mammals

These classes are all based on similarities. For instance all mammals have a similar skeleton, hair on their bodies, are warm bodied and suckle their young.

The class Mammalia (the mammals) contains 3 **subclasses**:

- Duck billed platypus and the spiny anteater
- **Marsupials** (animals like the kangaroo with pouches)
- **True mammals** (with a placenta)

Within the subclass containing the true mammals, there are groupings called **orders** that contain mammals that are more closely similar or related, than others. Examples of six mammalian orders are given below:

- Rodents (Rodentia) (rats and mice)
- Carnivores (Carnivora) (cats, dogs, bears and seals)
- Even-toed grazers (Artiodactyla) (pigs, sheep, cattle, antelopes)
- Odd-toed grazers (Perissodactyla) (horses, donkeys, zebras)
- Marine mammals (Cetacea) (whales, sea cows)
- Primates (monkeys, apes, humans)

Within each order there are various **families**. For example within the carnivore mammals are the families:

- Canidae (dog-like carnivores)
- Felidae (cat-like carnivores)

Even at this point it is possible to find groupings that are more closely related than others. These groups are called **genera** (singular genus). For instance within the cat family Felidae is the genus Felis containing the cats, as well as genera containing panthers, lynxes, and sabre toothed tigers!

The final groups within the system are the **species**. The definition of a species is a **group of animals that can mate successfully and produce fertile offspring**. This means that all domestic cats belong to the species *Felis domesticus*, because all breeds of cat whether Siamese, Manx or ordinary House hold cat can cross breed. However, domestic cats can not mate successfully with lions, tigers or jaguars, so these are placed in separate species, e.g. *Felis leo, Felis tigris and Felis onca.*

Even within the same species, there can be animals with quite wide variations in appearance that still breed successfully. We call these different **breeds, races** or **varieties**. For example there are many different breeds of dogs from Dalmatian to Chihuahua and of cats, from Siamese to Manx and domestic short-hairs, but all can cross breed. Often these breeds have been produced by **selective breeding** but varieties can arise in the wild when groups of animals are separated by a mountain range or sea and have developed different characteristics over long periods of time.

To summarise, the classification system consists of:

The **A**nimal **K**ingdom which is divided into

Phyla which are divided into

Classes which are divided into

Orders which are divided into

Families which are divided into

Genera which are divided into

Species.

"**Kings Play Cricket On Flat Green Surfaces**" OR "**Kindly Professors Cannot Often Fail Good Students**" are just two of the phrases students use to remind themselves of the order of these categories - on the other hand you might like to invent your own.

Summary

- The **scientific name** of an animal has two parts, the **genus** and the **species**, and must be written in **italics** or **underlined**.
- Animals are divided into **vertebrates** and **invertebrates**.
- The classification system has groupings called **phyla**, **classes**, **orders**, **families**, **genera** and **species**.
- Furry, milk-producing animals are all in the class **Mammalia.**
- Members within a **species** can mate and produce fertile offspring.
- Sub-groups within a species include **breeds, races** and **varieties**.

Worksheet

Work through the exercises in this Classification Worksheet [2] to help you learn how to write scientific names and classify different animals.

Test Yourself

1a) Re-write this scientific name for an animal correctly: trichosurus Vulpecula.

1b) Can you find out what this animal is?

2. Rearrange these groups from the biggest to the smallest:

   a) cars | diesel cars | motor vehicles | my diesel Toyota | transportation

   b) class | species | phylum | genus | order | kingdom | family | breed

3. Is a rabbit a rodent?

Test Yourself Answers

Websites

Classification

- http://www.mcwdn.org/Animals/AnimalClassQuiz.html Animal classification quiz

In fact much more than that. There is an elementary cell biology and classification quiz but the best thing about this website are the links to tables of characteristics of the different animal groups, for animals both with and without backbones.

- http://animaldiversity.ummz.umich.edu/site/index.html Animal diversity web

Careful! You could waste all day exploring this wonderful website. Chose an animal or group of animals you want to know about and you will see not only the classification but photos and details of distribution, behaviour and conservation status etc.

- http://www.indianchild.com/animal_kingdom.htm Indian child

Nice clear explanation of the different categories used in the classification of animals.

Glossary

- Link to Glossary [4]

References

[1] http://flickr.com/photos/grrphoto/307172203
[2] http://www.wikieducator.org/Classification_Worksheet

Anatomy and Physiology of Animals/Classification/Test Yourself Answers

1a) Re-write this scientific name for an animal correctly: trichosurus Vulpecula.

Trichosurus vulpecula or Trichosurus vulpecula

1b) Can you find out what this animal is?

The animal is a possum

2. Rearrange these groups from the biggest to the smallest:

a) cars | diesel cars | motor vehicles | my diesel Toyota | transportation

transportation | motor vehicles | cars | diesel cars | my diesel Toyota

b) class | species | phylum | genus | order | kingdom | family | breed

kingdom | phylum | class | order | family | genus | species | breed

3. Is a rabbit a rodent?

No – it is in the order Lagomorpha, not Rodentia. It is a lagomorph!

Anatomy and Physiology of Animals/The Cell

Objectives

After completing this section, you should know:

- that cells can be different shapes and sizes
- the role and function of the plasma membrane; cytoplasm, ribosomes, rough endoplasmic reticulum; smooth endoplasmic reticulum, mitochondria, golgi bodies, lysosomes, centrioles and the nucleus
- the structure of the plasma membrane
- that substances move across the plasma membrane by passive and active processes
- that passive processes include diffusion, osmosis and facilitated diffusion and active processes include active transport, pinocytosis, phagocytosis and exocytosis
- what the terms hypotonic, hypertonic isotonic and haemolysis mean
- that the nucleus contains the chromosomes formed from DNA
- that mitosis is the means by which ordinary cells divide
- the main stages of mitosis
- that meiosis is the process by which the chromosome number is halved when ova and sperm are formed

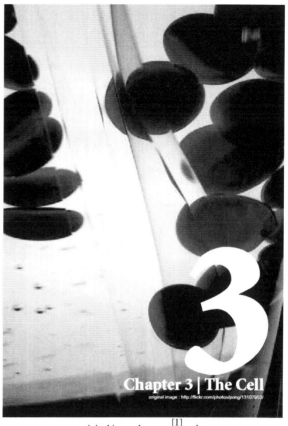

original image by pong [1] cc by

The Cell

The cell is the basic building block of living organisms. Bacteria and the parasite that causes malaria consist of single cells, while plants and animals are made up of trillions of cells. Most cells are spherical or cube shaped but some are a range of different shapes (see diagram 3.1).

Most cells are so small that a microscope is needed to see them, although a few cells, e.g. the ostrich's egg, are so large that they could make a meal for several people.

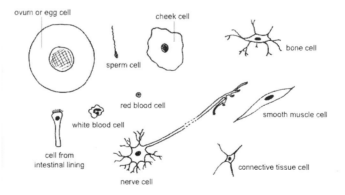

Diagram 3.1: A variety of animal cells

A normal cell is about 0.02 of a millimetre (0.02mm) in diameter. (Small distances like this are normally expressed in micrometres or microns (μm). Note there are 1000 μms in every mm).

When you look at a typical animal cell with a light microscope it seems quite simple with only a few structures visible (see diagram 3.2).

Three main parts can be seen:

- an outer cell wall or plasma membrane,
- an inner region called the cytoplasm and
- the nucleus

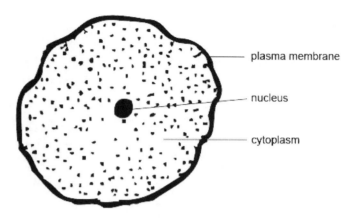

Diagram 3.2: An animal cell

However, when you use an electron microscope to increase the magnification many thousands of times you see that these seemingly simple structures are incredibly complex, each with its own specialized function. For example the plasma membrane is seen to be a double layer and the cytoplasm contains many special structures called **organelles** (meaning little organs) which are described below. A drawing of the cell as seen with an electron microscope is shown in diagram 3.3.

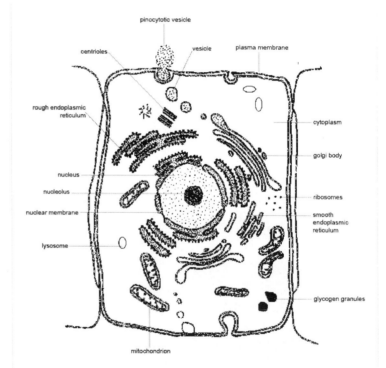

Diagram 3.3: An animal cell as seen with an electron microscope

The Plasma Membrane

The thin plasma membrane surrounds the cell, separating its contents from the surroundings and controlling what enters and leaves the cell. The plasma membrane is composed of two main molecules, fats (in fact phospholipids) and proteins. The fats are arranged in a double layer with the large protein molecules dotted about in the membrane (see diagram 3.4). Some of the protein molecules form tiny channels in the membrane while others help transport substances from one side of the membrane to the other.

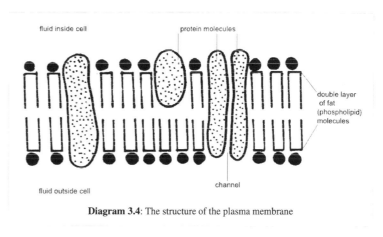

Diagram 3.4: The structure of the plasma membrane

How substances move across the Plasma Membrane

Substances need to pass through the membrane to enter or leave the cell and they do so in a number of ways. Some of these processes require no energy i.e. they are passive, while others require energy i.e. they are **active**.

Passive processes include: a) diffusion and b) osmosis, while active processes include: c) active transport, d) phagocytosis, e) pinocytosis and f) exocytosis. These will be described below.

a) Diffusion

Although you may not know it, you are already familiar with the process of diffusion. It is diffusion that causes a smell (expensive perfume or smelly socks) in one part of the room to gradually move through the room so it can be smelt on the other side. Diffusion occurs in the air and in liquids.

Diagram 3.5 shows what happens when a few crystals of a dark purple dye called potassium permanganate are dropped into a beaker of water. The dye molecules diffuse into the water moving from high to low concentrations so they become evenly distributed throughout the beaker.

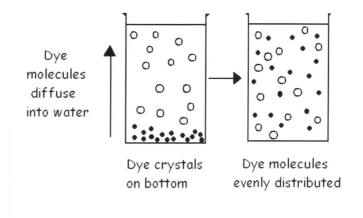

Diagram 3.5: Diffusion in a liquid

In the body, diffusion causes molecules that are in a high concentration on one side of the cell membrane to move across the membrane until they are present in equal concentrations on both sides. It takes place because all molecules have an in-built vibration that causes them to move and collide until they are evenly distributed. It is an absolutely natural process that requires no added energy.

Small molecules like oxygen, carbon dioxide, water and ammonia as well as fats, diffuse directly through the double fat layer of the membrane. The small molecules named above as well as a variety of charged particles (ions) also diffuse through the protein-lined channels. Larger molecules like glucose attach to a carrier molecule that aids their diffusion through the membrane. This is called **facilitated diffusion**.

In the animal's body diffusion is important for moving oxygen and carbon dioxide between the lungs and the blood, for moving digested food molecules from the gut into the blood and for the removal of waste products from the cell.

b) Osmosis

Although the word may be unfamiliar, you are almost certainly acquainted with the effects of osmosis. It is osmosis that plumps out dried fruit when you soak it before making a fruit cake or makes that wizened old carrot look almost like new when you soak it in water. Osmosis is in fact the diffusion of water across a membrane that allows water across but not larger molecules. This kind of membrane is called a **semi-permeable membrane**.

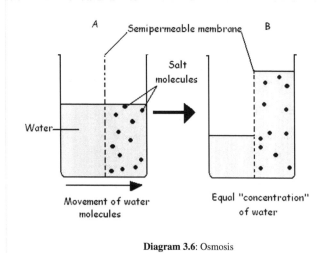

Diagram 3.6: Osmosis

Take a look at side **A** of diagram 3.6. It shows a container divided into two parts by an artificial semi-permeable membrane. Water is poured into one part while a solution containing salt is poured into the other part. Water can cross the membrane but the salt cannot. The water crosses the semi-permeable membrane by diffusion until there is an equal amount of water on both sides of the membrane. The effect of this would be to make the salt solution more diluted and cause the level of the liquid in the right-hand side of the container to rise so it looked like side **B** of diagram 3.6. This movement of water across the semi-permeable membrane is called osmosis. It is a completely natural process that requires no outside energy.

Although it would be difficult to do in practice, imagine that you could now take a plunger and push down on the fluid in the right-hand side of container **B** so that it flowed back across the semi-permeable membrane until the level of fluid on both sides was equal again. If you could measure the pressure required to do this, this would be equal to the **osmotic pressure** of the salt solution. (This is a rather advanced concept at this stage but you will meet this term again when you study fluid balance later in the course).

The plasma membrane of cells acts as a semi-permeable membrane. If red blood cells, for example, are placed in water, the water crosses the membrane to make the amount of water on both sides of it equal (see diagram 3.7). This means that the water moves into the cell causing it to swell. This can occur to such an extent that the cell actually bursts to release its contents. This bursting of red blood cells is called **haemolysis**. In a situation such as this when the solution on one side of a semi-permeable membrane has a lower concentration than that on the other side, the first solution is said to be **hypotonic** to the second.

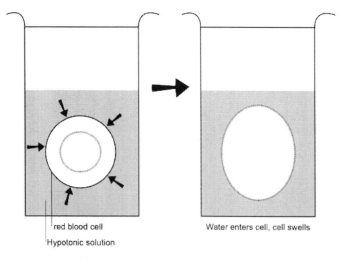

Diagram 3.7: Osmosis in red cells placed in a hypotonic solution

Now think what would happen if red blood cells were placed in a salt solution that has a higher salt concentration than the solution within the cells (see diagram 3.8). Such a bathing solution is called a **hypertonic** solution. In this situation the "concentration" of water within the cells would be higher than that outside the cells. Osmosis (diffusion of water) would then occur from the inside of the cells to the outside solution, causing the cells to shrink.

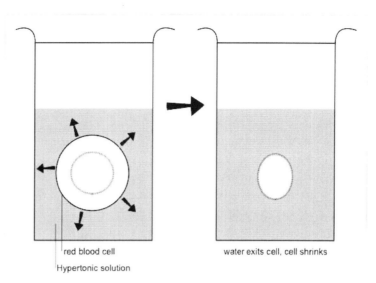

red blood cell

Hypertonic solution

water exits cell, cell shrinks

Diagram 3.8: Osmosis in red cells placed in a hypertonic solution

A solution that contains 0.9% salt has the same concentration as body fluids and the solution within red cells. Cells placed in such a solution would neither swell nor shrink (see diagram 3.9). This solution is called an **isotonic** solution. This strength of salt solution is often called **normal saline** and is used when replacing an animal's body fluids or when cells like red blood cells have to be suspended in fluid.

Remember - osmosis is a special kind of diffusion. It is the diffusion of water molecules across a semi-permeable membrane. It is a completely passive process and requires no energy.

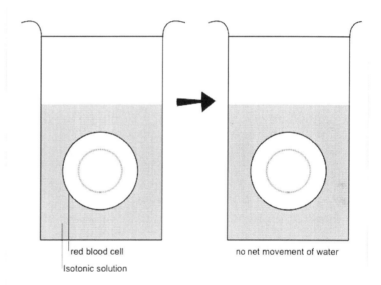

red blood cell

Isotonic solution

no net movement of water

Diagram 3.9: Red cells placed in an isotonic solution

Sometimes it is difficult to remember which way the water molecules move. Although it is not strictly true in a biological sense, many students use the phrase **"SALT SUCKS"** to help them remember which way water moves across the membrane when there are two solutions of different salt concentrations on either side.

As we have seen water moves in and out of the cell by osmosis. All water movement from the intestine into the blood system and between the blood capillaries and the fluid around the cells (tissue or extra cellular fluid) takes place by osmosis. Osmosis is also important in the production of concentrated urine by the kidney.

c) Active transport

When a substance is transported from a low concentration to a high concentration i.e. uphill against the concentration gradient, energy has to be used. This is called **active transport**.

Active transport is important in maintaining different concentrations of the ions sodium and potassium on either side of the nerve cell membrane. It is also important for removing valuable molecules such as glucose, amino acids and sodium ions from the urine.

d) Phagocytosis

Phagocytosis is sometimes called "cell eating". It is a process that requires energy and is used by cells to move solid particles like bacteria across the plasma membrane. Finger-like projections from the plasma membrane surround the bacteria and engulf them as shown in diagram 3.10. Once within the cell, enzymes produced by the lysosomes of the cell (described later) destroy the bacteria.

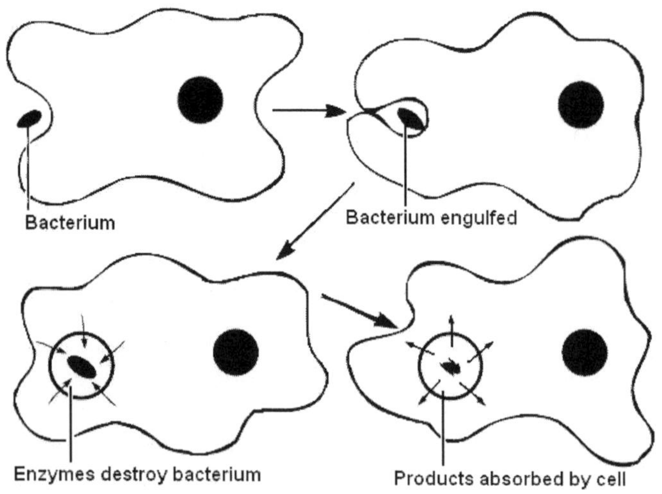

The destruction of bacteria and other foreign substance by white blood cells by the process of phagocytosis is a vital part of the defense mechanisms of the body.

Diagram 3.10: Phagocytosis

e) Pinocytosis

Pinocytosis or "cell drinking" is a very similar process to phagocytosis but is used by cells to move fluids across the plasma membrane. Most cells carry out pinocytosis (note the pinocytotic vesicle in diagram 3.3).

f) Exocytosis

Exocytosis is the process by means of which substances formed in the cell are moved through the plasma membrane into the fluid outside the cell (or extra-cellular fluid). It occurs in all cells but is most important in secretory cells (e.g. cells that produce digestive enzymes) and nerve cells.

The Cytoplasm

Within the plasma membrane is the **cytoplasm**. It consists of a clear jelly-like fluid called the a) **cytosol** or **intracellular fluid** in which b) **cell inclusions**, c) **organelles** and d) **microfilaments** and **microtubules** are found.

a) Cytosol

The cytosol consists mainly of water in which various molecules are dissolved or suspended. These molecules include proteins, fats and carbohydrates as well as sodium, potassium, calcium and chloride ions. Many of the reactions that take place in the cell occur in the cytosol.

b) Cell inclusions

These are large particles of fat, glycogen and melanin that have been produced by the cell. They are often large enough to be seen with the light microscope. For example the cells of adipose tissue (as in the insulating fat layer under the skin) contain fat that takes up most of the cell.

c) Organelles

Organelles are the "little organs" of the cell - like the heart, kidney and liver are the organs of the body. They are structures with characteristic appearances and specific "jobs" in the cell. Most can not be seen with the light microscope and so it was only when the electron microscope was developed that they were discovered. The main organelles in the cell are the **ribosomes, endoplasmic reticulum, mitochondrion, Golgi complex** and **lysosomes**. A cell containing these organelles as seen with the electron microscope is shown in diagram 3.3.

Ribosomes

Ribosomes are tiny spherical organelles that make proteins by joining amino acids together. Many ribosomes are found free in the cytosol, while others are attached to the rough endoplasmic reticulum.

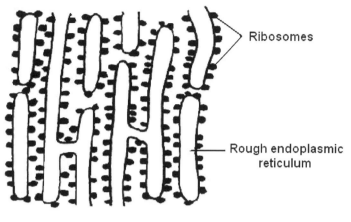

Endoplasmic reticulum

The **endoplasmic reticulum (ER)** is a network of membranes that form channels throughout the cytoplasm from the nucleus to the plasma membrane. Various molecules are made in the ER and transported around

Diagram 3.11: Rough endoplasmic reticulum

the cell in its channels. There are two types of ER: smooth ER and rough ER.

Smooth ER is where the fats in the cell are made and in some cells, where chemicals like alcohol, pesticides and carcinogenic molecules are inactivated.

The **Rough ER** has ribosomes attached to its surface. The function of the Rough ER is therefore to make proteins that are modified stored and transported by the ER (Diagram 3.11).

Mitochondria

Mitochondria (singular mitochondrion) are oval or rod shaped organelles scattered throughout the cytoplasm. They consist of two membranes, the inner one of which is folded to increase its surface area. (Diagram 3.12)

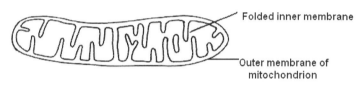

Diagram 3.12: A mitochondrion

Mitochondria are the "power stations" of the cell. They make energy by "burning" food molecules like glucose. This process is called **cellular respiration**. The reaction requires oxygen and produces carbon dioxide which is a waste product. The process is very complex and takes place in a large number of steps but the overall word equation for cellular respiration is-

Glucose + oxygen = carbon dioxide + water + energy

Note that cellular respiration is different from respiration or breathing. Breathing is the means by which air is drawn into and expelled from the lungs. Breathing is necessary to supply the cells with the oxygen required by the mitochondria and to remove the carbon dioxide produced as a waste product of cellular respiration.

Active cells like muscle, liver, kidney and sperm cells have large numbers of mitochondria.

Golgi Apparatus

The **Golgi bodies** in a cell together make up the **Golgi apparatus**. Golgi bodies are found near the nucleus and consist of flattened membranes stacked on top of each other rather like a pile of plates (see diagram 3.13). The Golgi apparatus modifies and sorts the proteins and fats made by the ER, then surrounds them in a membrane as **vesicles** so they can be moved to other parts of the cell.

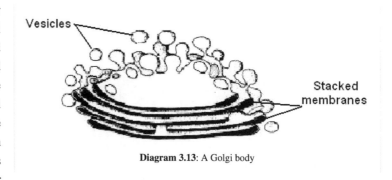

Diagram 3.13: A Golgi body

Lysosomes

Lysosomes are large vesicles that contain digestive enzymes. These break down bacteria and other substances that are brought into the cell by phagocytosis or pinocytosis. They also digest worn-out or damaged organelles, the components of which can then be recycled by the cell to make new structures.

d) Microfilaments And Microtubules

Some cells can move and change shape and organelles and chemicals are moved around the cell. Threadlike structures called **microfilaments** and **microtubules** that can contract are responsible for this movement.

These structures also form the projections from the plasma membrane known as **flagella** (singular flagellum) as in the sperm tail, and **cilia** found lining the respiratory tract and used to remove mucus that has trapped dust particles (see chapter 4).

Microtubules also form the pair of cylindrical structures called **centrioles** found near the nucleus. These help organise the spindle used in cell division.

The Nucleus

The **nucleus** is the largest structure in a cell and can be seen with the light microscope. It is a spherical or oval body that contains the **chromosomes**. The nucleus controls the development and activity of the cell. Most cells contain a nucleus although mature red blood cells have lost theirs during development and some muscle cells have several nuclei.

A double membrane similar in structure to the plasma membrane surrounds the nucleus (now called the nuclear envelope). Pores in this nuclear

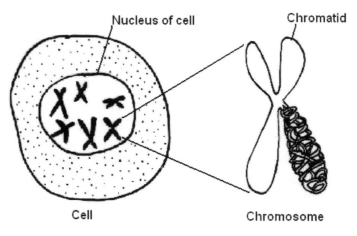

Diagram 3.14: A cell with an enlarged chromosome

membrane allow communication between the nucleus and the cytoplasm.

Within the nucleus one or more spherical bodies of darker material can be seen, even with the light microscope. These are called **nucleoli** and are made of RNA. Their role is to make new ribosomes.

Chromosomes

Inside the nucleus are the chromosomes which:

- contain DNA;
- control the activity of the cell;
- are transmitted from cell to cell when cells divide;
- are passed to a new individual when sex cells fuse together in sexual reproduction.

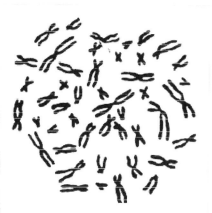

Diagram 3.15: A full set of human chromosomes

In cells that are not dividing the chromosomes are very long and thin and appear as dark grainy material. They become visible just before a cell divides when they shorten and thicken and can then be counted (see diagram 3.14).

The number of chromosomes in the cells of different species varies but is constant in the cells of any one species (e.g. horses have 64 chromosomes, cats have 38 and humans 46). Chromosomes occur in pairs (i.e. 32 pairs in the horse nucleus and 19 in that of the cat). Members of each pair are identical in length and shape and if you look carefully at diagram 3.15, you may be able to see some of the pairs in the human set of chromosomes.

Cell Division

Cells divide when an animal grows, when its body repairs an injury and when it produces sperm and eggs (or ova). There are two types of cell division: **Mitosis** and **meiosis**.

Mitosis. This is the cell division that occurs when an animal grows and when tissues are repaired or replaced. It produces two new cells (daughter cells) each with a full set of chromosomes that are identical to each other and to the parent cell. All the cells of an animal's body therefore contain identical DNA.

Meiosis. This is the cell division that produces the ova and sperm necessary for sexual reproduction. It only occurs in the ovary and testis.

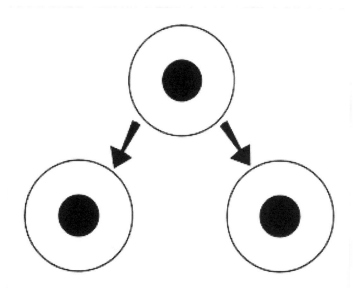

Diagram 3.16: Division by mitosis results in 2 new cells identical to each other and to parent cell

The most important function of meiosis it to halve the number of chromosomes so that when the sperm fertilises the ovum the normal number is regained. Body cells with the full set of chromosomes are called **diploid** cells, while **gametes** (sperm and ova) with half the chromosomes are called **haploid** cells.

Meiosis is a more complex process than mitosis as it involves two divisions one after the other and the four cells produced are all genetically different from each other and from the parent cell.

This fact that the cells formed by meiosis are all genetically different from each other and from the parent cell can be seen in litters of kittens where all the members of the litter are

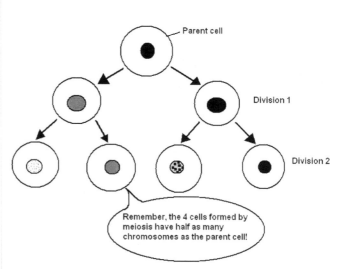

Diagram 3.17: Division by meiosis results in 4 new cells that are genetically different to each other

different from each other as well as being different from the parents although they display characteristics of both.

The Cell As A Factory

To make the function of the parts of the cell easier to understand and remember you can compare them to a factory. For example:

- The nucleus (1) is the managing director of the factory consulting the blueprint (the chromosomes) (2);
- The mitochondria (3) supply the power
- The ribosomes (4) make the products;
- The chloroplasts of plant cells (5) supply the fuel (food)
- The Golgi apparatus (6) packages the products ready for dispatch;
- The ER (7) modifies, stores and transports the products around the factory;
- The plasma membrane is the factory wall and the gates (8);
- The lysosomes dispose of the waste and worn-out machinery.

The cell compared to a factory [2]

Summary

- Cells consist of three parts: the **plasma membrane, cytoplasm** and **nucleus**.
- Substances pass through the plasma membrane by **diffusion** (gases, lipids), **osmosis** (water), **active transport** (glucose, ions), **phagocytosis** (particles), **pinocytosis** (fluids) and **exocytosis** (particles and fluids).
- **Osmosis** is the diffusion of **water** through a **semipermeable membrane**. Water diffuses from high water "concentration" to low water "concentration".
- The cytoplasm consists of **cytosol** in which are suspended **cell inclusions** and **organelles**.
- organelles include **ribosomes, endoplasmic reticulum, mitochondria, Golgi bodies** and **lysosomes**.
- The **nucleus** controls the activity of the cell. It contains the **chromosomes** that are composed of **DNA**.
- The cell divides by **mitosis** and **meiosis**

Worksheets

There are several worksheets you can use to help you understand and learn about the cell.

Plasma Membrane Worksheet [3]

Diffusion and Osmosis Worksheet 1 [4]

Diffusion and Osmosis Worksheet 2 [5]

Cell Division Worksheet [6]

Test Yourself

You can then test yourself to see how much you remember.

1. Complete the table below:

	Requires energy	Requires a semi permeable membrane?	Is the movement of water molecules only?	Molecules move from high to low concentration?	Molecules move from low to high concentration?
Diffusion	?	?	?	Yes	?
Osmosis	?	?	?	?	?
Active Transport	?	Yes	?	?	Yes

2. Red blood cells placed in a 5% salt solution would:

   swell/stay the same/ shrink?

3. Red blood cells placed in a 0.9% solution of salt would be in a:

   hypotonic/isotonic/hypertonic solution?

4. White blood cells remove foreign bodies like bacteria from the body by engulfing them. This process is known as

....

5. Match the organelle in the left hand column of the table below with its function in the right hand column.

Organelle	Function
a. Nucleus	1. Modifies proteins and fats
b. Mitochondrion	2. Makes, modifies and stores proteins
c. Golgi body	3. Digests worn out organelles
d. Rough endoplasmic reticulum	4. Makes fats
e. Lysosome	5. Controls the activity of the cell proteins
f. Smooth endoplasmic reticulum	6. Produces energy

6. The cell division that causes an organism to grow and repairs tissues is called:

7. The cell division that produces sperm and ova is called:

8. TWO important differences between the two types of cell division named by you above are:

   a.

   b.

Test Yourself Answers

Websites

- http://www.cellsalive.com/Cells alive

    Cells Alive gives good animations of the animal cell.

- Cell Wikipedia

    Wikipedia is good for almost anything you want to know about cells. Just watch as there is much more here than you need to know.

- http://personal.tmlp.com/Jimr57/textbook/chapter3/chapter3.htm Virtual cell

    The Virtual Cell has beautiful pictures of lots of (virtual?) cell organelles.

- http://www.wisc-online.com/objects/index_tj.asp?objid=AP11403 Typical animal cell

    Great interactive animal cell.

- http://www.wiley.com/college/apcentral/anatomydrill/Anatomy drill and practice

    Cell to test yourself on by dragging labels.

- http://www.maxanim.com/physiology/index.htm Max Animations

    Great animations here of diffusion, osmosis, facilitated diffusion, endo- and exocytosis and the development and action of lysosomes. A bit higher level than you need but still not to be missed.

- http://www.stolaf.edu/people/giannini/flashanimat/transport/diffusion.swf Diffusion

    Diffusion animation - good and clear.

- http://www.tvdsb.on.ca/westmin/science/sbi3a1/Cells/Osmosis.htm Osmosis

    Nice simple osmosis animation.

- http://zoology.okstate.edu/zoo_lrc/biol1114/tutorials/Flash/Osmosis_Animation.htm Osmosis

    Diffusion and osmosis. Watch what happens to the water and the solute molecules.

- http://www.wisc-online.com/objects/index_tj.asp?objid=NUR4004 Osmotic Pressure

    Do an online experiment to illustrate osmosis and osmotic pressure.

- http://www.stolaf.edu/people/giannini/flashanimat/transport/osmosis.swf Osmosis

    Even better osmosis demonstration - you get to add the salt.

Glossary

- Link to Glossary

References

[1] http://flickr.com/photos/pong/13107953/
[2] http://www.harunyahya.com/images_books/images_Dna/1.jpg
[3] http://www.wikieducator.org/Plasma_Membrane_Worksheet
[4] http://www.wikieducator.org/Diffusion_and_Osmosis_Worksheet_1
[5] http://www.wikieducator.org/Diffusion_and_Osmosis_Worksheet_2
[6] http://www.wikieducator.org/Cell_Division_Worksheet

Anatomy and Physiology of Animals/The Cell/Test Yourself Answers

1.

	Requires energy	Requires a semi permeable membrane?	Is the movement of water molecules only?	Molecules move from high to low concentration?	Molecules move from low to high concentration?
Diffusion	No	No	No	Yes	No
Osmosis	No	Yes	Yes	Yes	No
Active Transport	Yes	Yes	No	No	Yes

2. Red blood cells placed in a 5% salt solution would shrink as water flowed out of them into the hypertonic salt solution round them.

3. Red blood cells placed in a 0.9% solution of salt would be in an *isotonic solution*.

4. White blood cells remove foreign bodies like bacteria from the body by *phagocytosis*.

5.

Organelle	Function
a. Nucleus	5. Controls the activity of the cell
b. Mitochondrion	6. Produces energy
c. Golgi body	1. Modifies proteins and fats
d. Rough endoplasmic reticulum	2. Makes, modifies and stores proteins
e. Lysosome	3. Digests worn out organelles
f. Smooth endoplasmic reticulum	4. Makes fats

6. The cell division that causes an organism to grow and repairs tissues is called *mitosis*

7. The cell division that produces sperm and ova is called *meiosis*.

8. Two important differences between mitosis and meiosis are:

a) In mitosis the number of chromosomes in the cells formed is the same as in the original cell. In meiosis the number of chromosomes is halved.

b) In mitosis the cells formed are genetically identical to the original cell. In meiosis they are different.

Anatomy and Physiology of Animals/Body Organisation

In this chapter, the way the cells of the body are organised into different tissues is described. You will find out how these tissues are arranged into organs, and how the organs form systems such as the digestive system and the reproductive system. Also in this chapter, the important concept of homeostasis is defined. You are also introduced to those pesky things -- directional terms.

Objectives

After completing this section, you should know:

- the "Mrs Gren" characteristics of living organisms
- what a tissue is
- four basic types of tissues, their general function and where they are found in the body
- the basic organisation of the body of vertebrates including the main body cavities and the location of the following major organs: thorax, heart, lungs, thymus, abdomen, liver, stomach, spleen, intestines, kidneys, sperm ducts, ovaries, uterus, cervix, vagina, urinary bladder
- the 11 body systems
- what homeostasis is
- directional terms including dorsal, ventral, caudal, cranial, medial, lateral, proximal, distal, rostral, palmar and plantar. Plus transverse and longitudinal sections

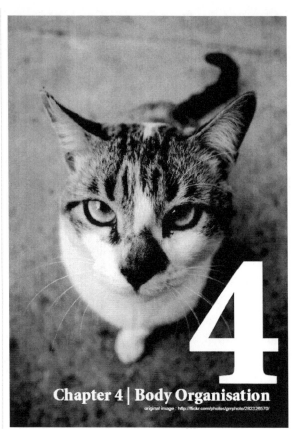

Chapter 4 | Body Organisation
original image : http://flickr.com/photos/grrphoto/282326570/

original image by grrphoto [1] cc by

The Organisation Of Animal Bodies

Living organisms move, feed, respire (burn food to make energy), grow, sense their environment, excrete and reproduce. These seven characteristics are sometimes summarized by the words "MRS GREN". functions of:

Movement

Respiration

Sensitivity

Growth

Reproduction

Excretion

Nutrition

Living organisms are made from cells which are organised into tissues and these are themselves combined to form organs and systems.

Skin cells, muscle cells, skeleton cells and nerve cells, for example. These different types of cells are not just scattered around randomly but similar cells that perform the same function are arranged in groups. These collections of similar cells are known as **tissues**.

There are four main types of tissues in animals. These are:

- **Epithelial** tissues that form linings, coverings and glands,
- **Connective** tissues for transport and support
- **Muscle** tissues for movement and
- **Nervous** tissues for carrying messages.

Epithelial Tissues

Epithelium (plural epithelia) is tissue that covers and lines. It covers an organ or lines a tube or space in the body. There are several different types of epithelium, distinguished by the different shapes of the cells and whether they consist of only a single layer of cells or several layers of cells.

Simple Epithelia - with a single layer of cells

Squamous epithelium

Squamous epithelium consists of a single layer of flattened cells that are shaped rather like 'crazy paving'. It is found lining the heart, blood vessels, lung alveoli and body cavities (see diagram 4.1). Its thinness allows molecules to diffuse across readily.

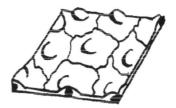

Diagram 4.1: Squamous epithelium

Cuboidal epithelium

Cuboidal epithelium consists of a single layer of cube shaped cells. It is rare in the body but is found lining kidney tubules (see diagram 4.2). Molecules pass across it by diffusion, osmosis and active transport.

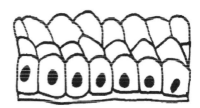

Diagram 4.2: Cuboidal epithelium

Columnar epithelium

Columnar epithelium consists of column shaped cells. It is found lining the gut from the stomach to the anus (see diagram 4.3). Digested food products move across it into the blood stream.

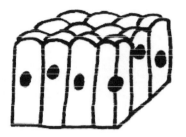

Diagram 4.3: Columnar epithelium

Columnar epithelium with cilia

Columnar epithelium with cilia on the free surface (also known as the apical side of the cell) lines the respiratory tract, fallopian tubes and uterus (see diagram 4.4). The cilia beat rhythmically to transport particles.

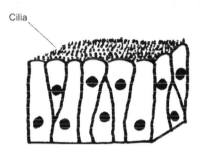

Diagram 4.4: Columnar epithelium with cilia

Transitional epithelium - with a variable number of layers

The cells in transitional epithelium can move over one another allowing it to stretch. It is found in the wall of the bladder (see diagram 4.5).

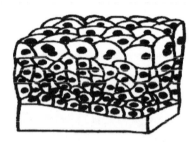

Diagram 4.5: Transitional epithelium

Stratified epithelia - with several layers of cells

Epithelia with several layers of cells are found where toughness and resistance to abrasion are needed.

Stratified squamous epithelium

Stratified squamous epithelium has many layers of flattened cells. It is found lining the mouth, cervix and vagina. Cells at the base divide and

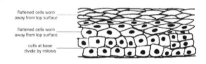

Diagram 4.6: Stratified squamous epithelium

push up the cells above them and cells at the top are worn or pushed off the surface (see diagram 4.6). This type of epithelium protects underlying layers and repairs itself rapidly if damaged.

Keratinised stratified squamous epithelium

Keratinised stratified squamous epithelium has a tough waterproof protein called **keratin** deposited in the cells. It forms the skin found covering the outer surface of mammals. (Skin will be described in more detail in Chapter 5).

Connective Tissues

Blood, bone, tendons, cartilage, fibrous connective tissue and fat (adipose) tissue are all classed as connective tissues. They are tissues that are used for supporting the body or transporting substances around the body. They also consist of three parts: they all have cells suspended in a ground substance or **matrix** and most have **fibres** running through it.

Blood

Blood consists of a matrix - plasma, with several types of cells and cell fragments suspended in it. The fibres are only evident in blood that has clotted. Blood will be described in detail in chapter 8.

Lymph

Lymph is similar in composition to blood plasma with various types of white blood cell floating in it. It flows in lymphatic vessels.

Connective tissue 'proper'

Connective tissue 'proper' consists of a jelly-like matrix with a dense network of collagen and elastic fibres and various cells embedded in it. There are various different forms of 'proper' connective tissue (see 1, 2 and 3 below).

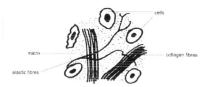

Diagram 4.7: Loose connective tissue

Loose connective tissue

Loose connective tissue is a sticky whitish substance that fills the spaces between organs. It is found in the dermis of the skin (see diagram 4.7).

Dense connective tissue

Dense connective tissue contains lots of thick fibres and is very strong. It forms tendons, ligaments and heart valves and covers bones and organs like the kidney and liver.

Adipose tissue

Adipose tissue consists of cells filled with fat. It forms the fatty layer under the dermis of the skin, around the kidneys and heart and the yellow marrow of the bones.

Cartilage

Cartilage is the 'gristle' of the meat. It consists of a tough jelly-like matrix with cells suspended in it. It may contain collagen and elastic fibres. It is a flexible but tough tissue and is found at the ends of bones, in the nose, ear and trachea and between the vertebrae (see diagram 4.8).

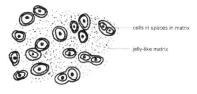

Diagram 4.8: Cartilage

Bone

Bone consists of a solid matrix made of calcium salts that give it its hardness. **Collagen** fibres running through it give it its strength. Bone cells are found in spaces in the matrix. Two types of bone are found in the skeleton namely **spongy** and **compact bone**. They differ in the way the cells and matrix are arranged. (See Chapter 6 for more details of bone).

Muscle Tissues

Muscle tissue is composed of cells that contract and move the body. There are three types of muscle tissue:

Smooth muscle

Smooth muscle consists of long and slender cells with a central nucleus (see diagram 4.9). It is found in the walls of blood vessels, airways to the lungs and the gut. It changes the size of the blood vessels and helps move food and fluid along. Contraction of smooth muscle fibres occurs without the conscious control of the animal.

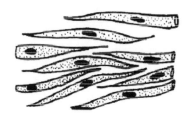

Diagram 4.9: Smooth muscle fibres

Skeletal muscle

Skeletal muscle (sometimes called **striated**, **striped** or **voluntary muscle**) has striped fibres with alternating light and dark bands. It is attached to bones and is under the voluntary control of the animal (see diagram 4.10).

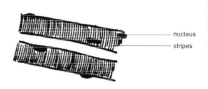

Diagram 4.10: Skeletal muscle fibres

Cardiac muscle

Cardiac muscle is found only in the walls of the heart where it produces the 'heart beat'. Cardiac muscle cells are branched cylinders with central nuclei and faint stripes (see diagram 4.11). Each fibre contracts automatically but the heart beat as a whole is controlled by the **pacemaker** and the involuntary **autonomic nervous system**.

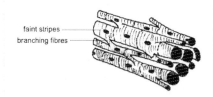

Diagram 4.11: Cardiac muscle fibres

Nervous Tissues

Nervous tissue forms the nerves, spinal cord and brain. Nerve cells or **neurons** consist of a cell body and a long thread or axon that carries the nerve impulse. An insulating sheath of fatty material (**myelin**) usually surrounds the axon. Diagram 4.12 shows a typical motor neuron that sends messages to muscles to contract.

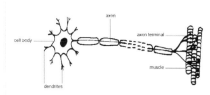

Diagram 4.12: A motor neuron

Vertebrate Bodies

We are so familiar with animals with backbones (i.e. vertebrates) that it seems rather unnecessary to point out that the body is divided into three sections. There is a well-defined **head** that contains the brain, the major sense organs and the mouth, a **trunk** that contains the other organs and a well-developed **tail**. Other features of vertebrates may be less apparent. For instance, vertebrates that live on the land have developed a flexible neck that is absent in fish where it would be in the way of the gills and interfere with streamlining. Mammals but not other vertebrates have a sheet of muscle called the **diaphragm** that divides the trunk into the chest region or **thorax** and the **abdomen**.

Body Cavities

In contrast to many primitive animals, vertebrates have spaces or **body cavities** that contain the body organs. Most vertebrates have a single body cavity but in mammals the diaphragm divides the main cavity into a **thoracic** and an **abdominal cavity**. In the thoracic cavity the heart and lungs are surrounded by their own membranes so that cavities are created around the heart - the **pericardial cavity**, and around the lungs – the **pleural cavity** (see diagram 4.13).

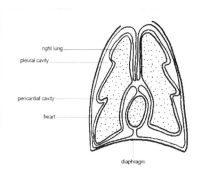

Diagram 4.13: The body cavities

Organs

Just as the various parts of the cell work together to perform the cell's functions and a large number of similar cells make up a tissue, so many different tissues can "cooperate" to form an organ that performs a particular function. For example, connective tissues, epithelial tissues, muscle tissue and nervous tissue combine to make the organ that we call the stomach. In turn the stomach combines with other organs like the intestines, liver and pancreas to form the digestive system (see diagram 4.14).

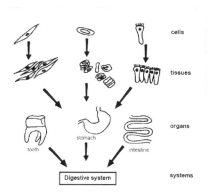

Diagram 4.14: Cells, tissues and organs forming the digestive system

Generalised Plan Of The Mammalian Body

At this point it would be a good idea to make yourself familiar with the major organs and their positions in the body of a mammal like the rabbit. Diagram 4.15 shows the main body organs.

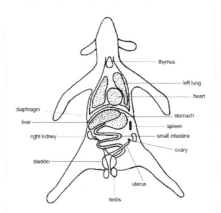

Diagram 4.15: The main organs of the vertebrate body

Body Systems

Organs do not work in isolation but function in cooperation with other organs and body structures to bring about the MRS GREN functions necessary to keep an animal alive. For example the stomach can only work in conjunction with the mouth and oesophagus (gullet). These provide it with the food it breaks down and digests. It then needs to pass the food on to the intestines etc. for further digestion and absorption. The organs involved with the taking of food into the body, the digestion and absorption of the food and elimination of waste products are collectively known as the digestive system.

The 11 body systems

1. Skin

    The skin covering the body consists of two layers, the **epidermis** and **dermis**. Associated with these layers are hairs, feathers, claws, hoofs, glands and sense organs of the skin.

2. Skeletal System

    This can be divided into the bones of the skeleton and the joints where the bones move over each other.

3. Muscular System

    The muscles, in conjunction with the skeleton and joints, give the body the ability to move.

4. Cardiovascular System

    This is also known as the circulatory system. It consists of the heart, the blood vessels and the blood. It transports substances around the body.

5. Lymphatic System

    This system is responsible for collecting and "cleaning" the fluid that leaks out of the blood vessels. This fluid is then returned to the blood system. The lymphatic system also makes antibodies that protect the body from invasion by bacteria etc. It consists of lymphatic vessels, lymph nodes, the spleen and thymus glands.

6. Respiratory System

    This is the system involved with bringing oxygen in the air into the body and getting rid of carbon dioxide, which is a waste product of processes that occur in the cell. It is made up of the trachea, bronchi, bronchioles, lungs, diaphragm, ribs and muscles that move the ribs in breathing.

7. Digestive System

    This is also known as the **gastrointestinal system**, **alimentary system** or **gut**. It consists of the digestive tube and glands like the liver and pancreas that produce digestive secretions. It is concerned with breaking down the large molecules in foods into smaller ones that can be absorbed into the blood and lymph. Waste material is also eliminated by the digestive system.

8. Urinary System

    This is also known as the **renal system**. It removes waste products from the blood and is made up of the kidneys, ureters and bladder.

9. Reproductive System

This is the system that keeps the species going by making new individuals. It is made up of the ovaries, uterus, vagina and fallopian tubes in the female and the testes with associated glands and ducts in the male.

10. Nervous System

This system coordinates the activities of the body and responses to the environment. It consists of the sense organs (eye, ear, semicircular canals, and organs of taste and smell), the nerves, brain and spinal cord.

11. Endocrine System

This is the system that produces chemical messengers or hormones. It consists of various **endocrine glands** (ductless glands) that include the pituitary, adrenal, thyroid and pineal glands as well as the testes and ovary.

Homeostasis

All the body systems, except the reproductive system, are involved with keeping the conditions inside the animal more or less stable. This is called **homeostasis**. These constant conditions are essential for the survival and proper functioning of the cells, tissues and organs of the body. The skin, for example, has an important role in keeping the temperature of the body constant. The kidneys keep the concentration of salts in the blood within limits and the islets of Langerhans in the pancreas maintain the correct level of glucose in the blood through the hormone insulin. As long as the various body processes remain within normal limits, the body functions properly and is healthy. Once homeostasis is disturbed disease or death may result. (See Chapters 12 and 16 for more on homeostasis).

Directional Terms

In the following chapters the systems of the body in the list above will be covered one by one. For each one the structure of the organs involved will be described and the way they function will be explained.

In order to describe structures in the body of an animal it is necessary to have a system for describing the position of parts of the body in relation to other parts. For example it may be necessary to describe the position of the liver in relation to the diaphragm, or the heart in relation to the lungs. Certainly if you work further with animals, in a veterinary clinic for example, it will be necessary to be able to accurately describe the position of an injury. The terms used for this are called **directional terms**.

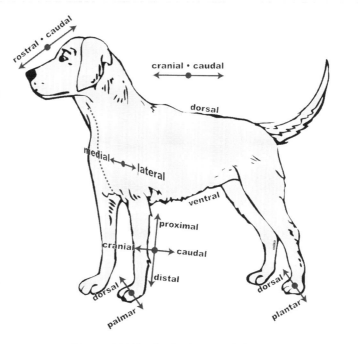

Diagram 4.16: The directional terms used with animals

The most common directional terms are **right** and **left**. However, even these are not completely straightforward especially when looking at diagrams of animals. The convention is to show the left side of the animal or organ on the right side of the page. This is the view you would get looking down on an animal lying on its back during surgery or in a post-mortem. Sometimes it is useful to imagine 'getting inside' the animal (so to speak) to check which side is which. The other common and useful directional terms are listed below and shown in diagram 4.16.

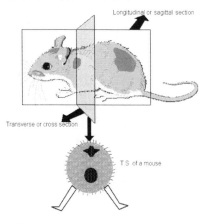

Diagram 4.17: Transverse and longitudinal sections of a mouse

Term	Definition	Example
Dorsal	Nearer the back of the animal than	The backbone is dorsal to the belly
Ventral	Nearer the belly of the animal than	The breastbone is ventral to the heart
Cranial (or anterior)	Nearer to the skull than	The diaphragm is cranial to the stomach
Caudal (or posterior)	Nearer to the tail than	The ribs are caudal to the neck
Proximal	Closer to the body than (only used for structures on limbs)	The shoulder is proximal to the elbow
Distal	Further from the body than (only used for structures on limbs)	The ankle is distal to the knee
Medial	Nearer to the midline than	The bladder is medial to the hips
Lateral	Further from the midline than	The ribs are lateral to the lungs
Rostral	Towards the muzzle	There are more grey hairs in the rostral part of the head
Palmar	The "walking" surface of the front paw	There is a small cut on the left palmar surface
Plantar	The "walking" surface of the hind paw	The pads are on the plantar side of the foot

Note that we don't use the terms **superior** and **inferior** for animals. They are only used to describe the position of structures in the human body (and possibly apes) where the upright posture means some structures are above or superior to others.

In order to look at the structure of some of the parts or organs of the body it may be necessary to cut them open or even make thin slices of them that they can be examined under the microscope. The direction and position of slices or sections through an animal's body have their own terminology.

If an animal or organ is sliced lengthwise this section is called a **longitudinal** or **sagittal section**. This is sometimes abbreviated to LS.

If the section is sliced crosswise it is called a **transverse** or **cross section**. This is sometimes abbreviated to TS or XS (see diagram 4.17).

Summary

- The characteristics of living organisms can be summarised by the words "**MRS GREN.**"
- There are 4 main types of tissue namely: **epithelial, connective, muscle** and **nervous tissues**.
- **Epithelial tissues** form the skin and line the gut, respiratory tract, bladder etc.
- **Connective tissues** form tendons, ligaments, adipose tissue, blood, cartilage and bone, and are found in the dermis of the skin.
- **Muscular tissues** contract and consist of 3 types: **smooth, skeletal and cardiac.**
- Vertebrate bodies have a **head, trunk** and **tail**. Body organs are located in **body cavities**. 11 body systems perform essential body functions most of which maintain a stable environment or **homeostasis** within the animal.
- **Directional terms** describe the location of parts of the body in relation to other parts.

Worksheets

Students often find it hard learning how to use directional terms correctly. There are two worksheets to help you with these and another on tissues.

Directional Terms Worksheet 1 [2]

Directional Terms Worksheet 2 [3]

Tissues Worksheet [4]

Test Yourself

1. Living organisms can be distinguished from non-living matter because they usually move and grow. Name 5 other functions of living organisms:

    1.

    2.

    3.

    4.

    5.

2. What tissue types would you find...

    a) lining the intestine:

    b) covering the body:

    c) moving bones:

    d) flowing through blood vessels:

    e) linking the eye to the brain:

    f) lining the bladder:

3. Name the body cavity in which the following organs are found:

    a) heart:

    b) bladder:

    c) stomach:

    d) lungs:

4. Name the body system that...

    a) includes the bones and joints:

    b) includes the ovaries and testes:

c) produces hormones:

d) includes the heart, blood vessels and blood:

5. What is homeostasis?

6. Circle which is correct:

a) The head is cranial | caudal to the neck

b) The heart is medial | lateral to the ribs

c) The elbow is proximal | distal to the fingers

d) The spine is dorsal | ventral to the heart

7. Indicate whether or not these statements are true.

a) The stomach is cranial to the diaphragm - true | false

b) The heart lies in the pelvic cavity - true | false

c) The spleen is roughly the same size as the stomach and lies near it - true | false

d) The small intestine is proximal to the kidneys - true | false

e) The bladder is medial to the hips - true | false

f) The liver is cranial to the heart - true | false

Test Yourself Answers

Websites

• Connective tissue

A fabulous site showing you actual photos of microscope sections of the different tissues with short explanations of each and even quizzes.

http://nhscience.lonestar.edu/BIOL/tissue.html

• Animal organ systems and homeostasis

Overview of the different organ systems (in humans) and their functions in maintaining homeostasis in the body.

http://www.emc.maricopa.edu/faculty/farabee/biobk/BioBookANIMORGSYS.html

• Wikipedia

Directional terms for animals. A little more detail than required but still great.

http://en.wikipedia.org/wiki/Anatomical_terms_of_location

Glossary

• Link to Glossary [4]

References

[1]   http://flickr.com/photos/grrphoto/282326570/
[2]   http://www.wikieducator.org/Directional_Terms_Worksheet_1
[3]   http://www.wikieducator.org/Directional_Terms_Worksheet_2
[4]   http://www.wikieducator.org/Tissues_Worksheet

Anatomy and Physiology of Animals/Body Organisation/Test Yourself Answers

1. Living organisms can be distinguished from non-living matter because *they usually move* and grow. They also excrete, respire, are sensitive to the environment, reproduce and feed. 2. What tissue types would you find:

a) *Columnar epithelial tissue* lines the intestine.

b) *Keratinised stratified squamous epithelium* covers the body.

c) *Skeletal muscle* moves bones.

d) *Blood* (a type of connective tissue) flows through blood vessels.

e) *Nerves* link the eye to the brain

f) *Transitional epithelium* lines the bladder

3. Name the body cavity in which the following organs are found:

a) The heart is located in the *pericardial cavity* (situated in the thoracic cavity).

b) The bladder is situated in the *pelvic cavity*

c) The stomach is situated in the *abdominal cavity*

d) The lungs are situated in the *pleural cavity* (also situated in the thoracic cavity).

4. Body systems

a) The *skeletal system* includes the bones and joints

b) The *reproductive system* includes the ovaries and testes

c) The *endocrine system* produces hormones.

d) The *circulatory system* includes the heart, blood vessels and blood.

5. Homeostasis is the *maintenance of constant conditions in an animal's body.*

6. Circle which is correct:

a) The head is *cranial* to the neck

b) The heart is *medial* to the ribs

c) The elbow is *proximal* to the fingers

d) The spine is *dorsal* to the heart

7. Indicate whether or not these statements are true.

a) The stomach is cranial to the diaphragm - *false. It is caudal to the diaphragm.*

b) The heart lies in the pelvic cavity - *false. It lies in the thoracic cavity or to be more precise in the pleural cavity.*

c) The spleen is roughly the same size as the stomach and lies near it - *true*

d) The small intestine is proximal to the kidneys - *false (remember the term proximal is only used when describing the relationship of parts of the limbs to each other). Perhaps it would be better to say that the small intestine is ventral to the kidneys.*

e) The bladder is medial to the hips - *true*

f) The liver is cranial to the heart - false. *The liver is caudal to the heart.*

Anatomy and Physiology of Animals/The Skin

The skin is the first of the eleven body systems to be described. Each chapter from now on will cover one body system.

The skin, sometimes known as the **Integumentary System** is, in fact, the largest organ of the body. It has a complex structure, being composed of many different tissues. It performs many functions that are important in maintaining homeostasis in the body. Probably the most important of these functions is the control of body temperature. The skin also protects the body from physical damage and bacterial invasion. The skin has an array of sense organs which sense the external environment, and also cells which can make **vitamin D** in sunlight.

The skin is one of the first systems affected when an animal becomes sick so it is important for anyone working with animals to have a sound knowledge of the structure and functioning of the skin so they can quickly recognise signs of disease.

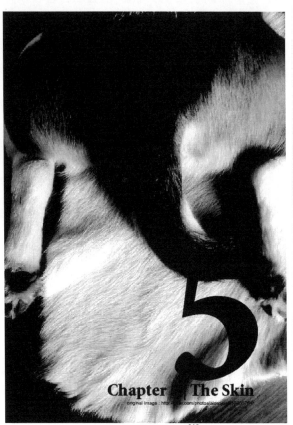

original image by Fran-cis-ca [1] cc by

Objectives

After completing this section, you should know:

- the general structure of the skin
- the function of the keratin deposited in the epidermis
- the structure and function of keratin skin structures including calluses, scales, nails, claws, hoofs and horns
- that antlers are not made either of keratin or in the epidermis
- the structure of hairs
- the structure of the different types of feathers and the function of preening
- the general structure and function of sweat, scent, preen and mammary glands
- the basic functions of the skin in sensing stimuli, temperature control and production of vitamin D
- the mechanisms by which the skin regulates body temperature

The Skin

Skin comes in all kinds of textures and forms. There is the dry warty skin of toads and crocodiles, the wet slimy skin of fish and frogs, the hard shell of tortoises and the soft supple skin of snakes and humans. Mammalian skin is covered with hair, that of birds with feathers, and fish and reptiles have scales. Pigment in the skin, hairs or feathers can make the outer surface almost any colour of the rainbow.

As humans, it is often the skin of an animal that gives it its appeal to us or repels us. We love the soft feel of a cat's coat but perhaps can't bear to touch a snake. As the main part of an animal visible to us, the skin can often give us clues to the health of an animal. A healthy animal will have a clean, glowing, flexible skin, while ill health may show itself as an abnormal colour or texture.

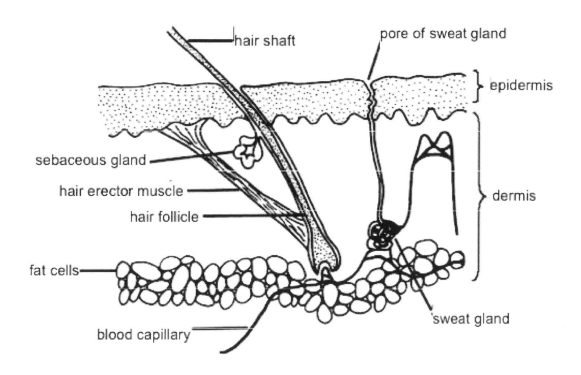

Diagram 5.1 - Cross section through the skin

Skin is one of the largest organs of the body, making up 6-8% of the total body weight. It consists of two distinct layers. The top layer is called the **epidermis** and under that is the **dermis** (see diagram 5.1).

The epidermis is the layer that bubbles up when we have a blister and as we know from this experience, it has no blood or nerves in it. The cells at the base of the epidermis continually divide and push the cells above them upwards. As these cells move up they die and become the dry flaky scales that fall off the skin surface. The cells in the epidermis die because a special protein called **keratin** is deposited in them. Keratin is an extremely important substance for it makes the skin waterproof. Without it land vertebrates like reptiles, birds and mammals would, like frogs, be able to survive only in damp places.

Skin Structures Made Of Keratin

Claws, Nails and Hoofs

Reptiles, birds and mammals all have nails or claws on the ends of their toes. They protect the end of the toe and may be used for grasping, grooming, digging or in defense. They are continually worn away and grow continuously from a growth layer at their base (see diagram 5.2).

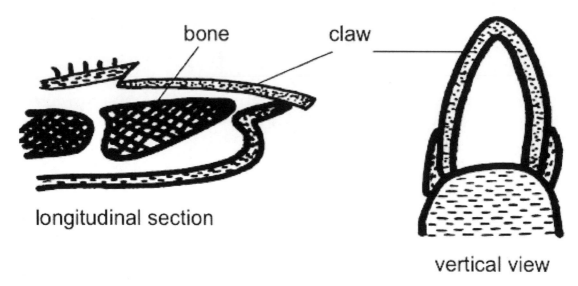

Diagram 5.2 - A carnivore's claw

Hoofs are found in sheep, cows, horses etc. otherwise known as **ungulate mammals**. These are animals that have lost toes in the process of evolution and walk on the "nails" of the remaining toes. The hoof is a cylinder of horny material that surrounds and protects the tip of the toe (see diagram 5.3).

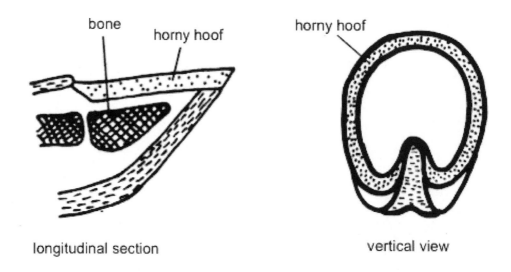

Diagram 5.3 - A horse's hoof

Horns And Antlers

True horns are made of keratin and are found in sheep, goats and cattle. They are never branched and, once grown, are never shed. They consist of a core of bone arising in the dermis of the skin and are fused with the skull. The horn itself forms as a hollow cone-shaped sheath around the bone (see diagram 5.4).

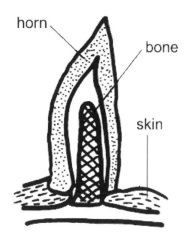

Diagram 5.4 - A horn

The **antlers** of male deer have quite a different structure. They are not formed in the epidermis and do not consist of keratin but are entirely of bone. They are shed each year and are often branched, especially in older animals. When growing they are covered in skin called **velvet** that forms the bone. Later the velvet is shed to leave the bony antler. The velvet is often removed artificially to be sold in Asia as a traditional medicine (see diagram 5.5).

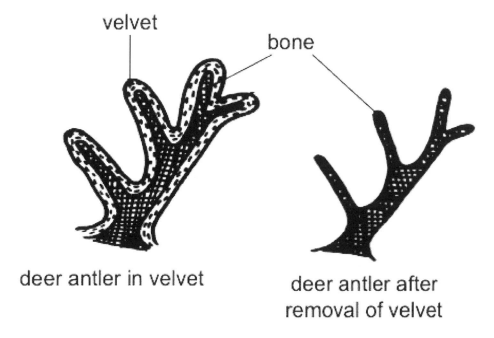

deer antler in velvet

deer antler after
removal of velvet

Diagram 5.5 - A deer antler

Other animals have projections on their heads that are not true horns either. The horns on the head of giraffes are made of bone covered with skin and hair, and the 'horn' of a rhinoceros is made of modified and fused hair-like structures.

Hair

Hair is also made of keratin and develops in the epidermis. It covers the body of most mammals where it acts as an insulator and helps to regulate the temperature of the body (see below). The colour in hairs is formed from the same pigment, **melanin** that colours the skin. Coat colour may help camouflage animals and sometimes acts to attract the opposite sex.

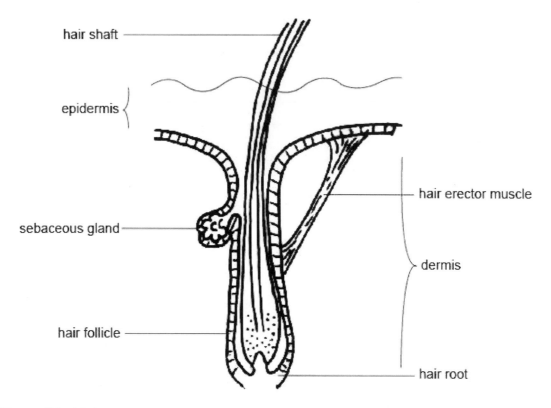

Diagram 5.6 - A hair

Hairs lie in a **follicle** and grow from a **root** that is well supplied with blood vessels. The hair itself consists of layers of dead keratin - containing cells and usually lies at a slant in the skin. A small bundle of smooth muscle fibres (the **hair erector muscle**) is attached to the side of each hair and when this contracts the hair stands on end. This increases the insulating power of the coat and is also used by some animals to make them seem larger when confronted by a foe or a competitor(see diagram 5.6).

The whiskers of cats and the spines of hedgehogs are examples of special types of hairs.

Feathers

The lightness and stiffness of keratin is also a key to bird flight. In the form of feathers it provides the large airfoils necessary for flapping and gliding flight. In another form, the light fluffy down feathers,also made of keratin, are some of the best natural insulators known. This superior insulation is necessary to help maintain the high body temperatures of birds.

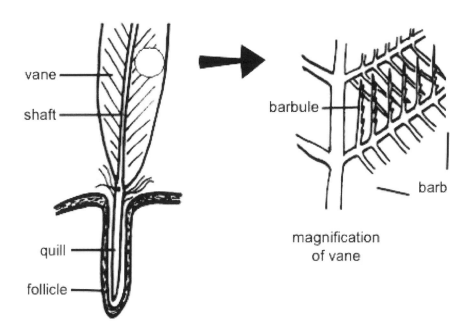

Diagram 5.7 - A Contour Feather

Countour feathers are large feathers that cover the body, wings and tail. They have an expanded **vane** that provides the smooth, continuous surface that is required for effective flight. This surface is formed by **barbs** that extend out from the central shaft. If you look carefully at a feather you can see that on either side of each barb are thousands of **barbules** that lock together by a complex system of hooks and notches. if this arrangement becomes disrupted, the bird uses its beak to draw the barbs and barbules together again in an action known as **preening** (see diagram 5.7).

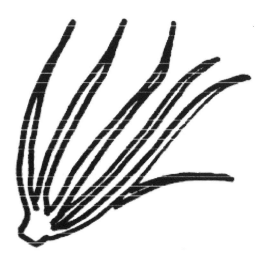

Diagram 5.8 - A Down Feather

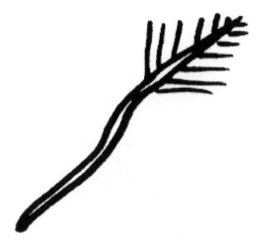

Diagram 5.9 - A Pin Feather

Down feathers are the only feathers covering a chick and form the main insulation layer under the contour feathers of the adult. They have no shaft but consist of a spray of simple, slender branches (see diagram 5.8).

Pin feathers have a slender hair-like shaft often with a tiny tuft of barbs on the end. They are found between the other feathers and help tell a bird how its feathers are lying (see diagram 5.9).

Skin Glands

Glands are organs that produce and secrete fluids. They are usually divided into two groups depending upon whether or not they have channels or ducts to carry their products away. Glands with ducts are called **exocrine glands** and include the glands found in the skin as well as the glands that produce digestive enzymes in the gut. **Endocrine glands** have no ducts and release their products (hormones) directly into the blood stream. The pituitary and adrenal glands are examples of endocrine glands.

Most vertebrates have exocrine glands in the skin that produce a variety of secretions. The slime on the skin of fish and frogs is **mucus** produced by skin glands and some fish and frogs also produce poison from modified glands. In fact the skin glands of some frogs produce the most poisonous chemicals known. Reptiles and birds have a dry skin with few glands. The **preen gland**, situated near the base of the bird's tail, produces oil to help keep the feathers in good condition. Mammals have an array of different skin glands. These include the wax producing, sweat, sebaceous and mammary glands.

Wax producing glands are found in the ears.

Sebaceous glands secrete an oily secretion into the hair follicle. This secretion, known as **sebum**, keeps the hair supple and helps prevent the growth of bacteria (see diagram 5.6).

Sweat glands consist of a coiled tube and a duct leading onto the skin surface. Their appearance when examined under the microscope inspired one of the first scientists to observe them to call them "fairies' intestines" (see diagram 5.1). Sweat contains salt and waste products like urea and the evaporation of sweat on the skin surface is one of the major mechanisms for cooling the body of many mammals. Horses can sweat up to 30 litres of fluid a day during active exercise, but cats and dogs have few sweat glands and must cool themselves by panting. Scent in the sweat of many animals is used to mark territory or attract the opposite sex.

Mammary glands are only present in mammals. They are thought to be modified sebaceous glands and are present in both sexes but are rarely active in males (see diagram 5.10). The number of glands varies from species to species. They open to the surface in well-developed nipples. Milk contains proteins, sugars, fats and salts, although the exact composition varies from one species to another.

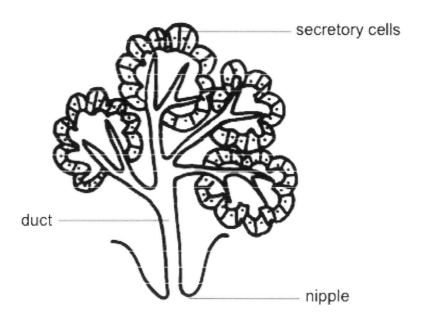

Diagram 5.10 - A Mammary Gland

The Skin And Sun

A moderate amount of UV in sunlight is necessary for the skin to form **vitamin D**. This vitamin prevents bone disorders like rickets to which animals reared indoors are susceptible. Excessive exposure to the UV in sunlight can be damaging and the pigment **melanin**, deposited in cells at the base of the epidermis, helps to protect the underlying layers of the skin from this damage. Melanin also colours the skin and variations in the amount of melanin produces colours from pale yellow to black.

Sunburn And Skin Cancer

Excess exposure to the sun can cause sunburn. This is common in humans, but light skinned animals like cats and pigs can also be sunburned, especially on the ears. Skin cancer can also result from excessive exposure to the sun. As holes in the ozone layer increase exposure to the sun's UV rays, so too does the rate of skin cancer in humans and animals.

The Dermis

The underlying layer of the skin, known as the dermis, is much thicker but much more uniform in structure than the epidermis (see diagram 5.1). It is composed of loose connective tissue with a felted mass of **collagen** and **elastic fibres**. It is this part of the skin of cattle and pigs etc. that becomes commercial leather when treated,. The dermis is well supplied with blood vessels, so cuts and burns that penetrate down into the dermis will bleed or cause serious fluid loss. There are also numerous nerve endings and touch receptors in the dermis because, of course, the skin is sensitive to touch, pain and temperature.

When looking at a section of the skin under the microscope you can see hair follicles, sweat and sebaceous glands dipping down into the dermis. However, these structures do not originate in the dermis but are derived from the epidermis.

In the lower levels of the dermis is a layer of fat or **adipose tissue** (see diagram 5.1). This acts as an energy store and is an excellent insulator especially in mammals like whales with little hair.

The Skin And Temperature Regulation

Vertebrates can be divided into two groups depending on whether or not they control their internal temperature. Amphibia (frogs) and reptiles are said to be "**cold blooded**" (**poikilothermic**) because their body temperature approximately follows that of the environment. Birds and mammals are said to be **warm blooded (homoiothermic)** because they can maintain a roughly constant body temperature despite changes in the temperature of the environment.

Heat is produced by the biochemical reactions of the body (especially in the liver) and by muscle contraction. Most of the heat lost from the body occurs via the skin. It is therefore not surprising that many of the mechanisms for controlling the temperature of the body operate here.

Reduction Of Heat Loss

When an animal is in a cold environment and needs to reduce heat loss the erector muscles contract causing the hair or feathers to rise up and increase the layer of insulating air trapped by them (see diagram 5.11a).

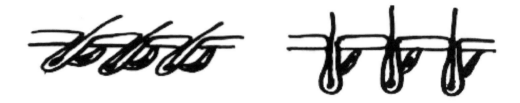

Diagram 5.11a) Hair muscle relaxed...............Diagram 5.11b) Hair muscle contracted

Heat loss from the skin surface can also be reduced by the contraction of the abundant blood vessels that lie in the dermis. This takes blood flow to deeper levels, so reducing heat loss and causing pale skin (see diagram 5.12a).

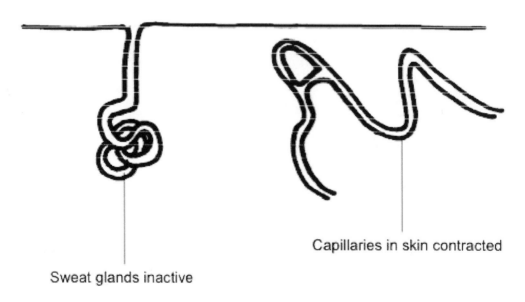

Capillaries in skin contracted

Sweat glands inactive

Diagram 5.12a) Reduction of heat loss by skin

Shivering caused by twitching muscles produces heat that also helps raise the body temperature.

Increase Of Heat Loss

There are two main mechanisms used by animals to increase the amount of heat lost from the skin when they are in a hot environment or high levels of activity are increasing internal heat production. The first is the expansion of the blood vessels in the dermis so blood flows near the skin surface and heat loss to the environment can take place. The second is by the production of sweat from the sweat glands (see diagram 5.12b). The evaporation of this liquid on the skin surface produces a cooling effect.

The mechanisms for regulating body temperature are under the control of a small region of the brain called the **hypothalamus**. This acts like a thermostat.

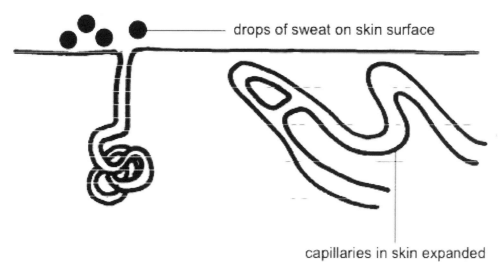

Diagram 5.12b) - Increase of heat loss by skin

Heat Loss And Body Size

The amount of heat that can be lost from the surface of the body is related to the area of skin an animal has in relation to the total volume of its body.

Small animals like mice have a very large skin area compared to their total volume. This means they tend to loose large amounts of heat and have difficulty keeping warm in cold weather. They may need to keep active just to maintain their body temperature or may hibernate to avoid the problem.

Large animals like elephants have the opposite problem. They have only a relatively small skin area in relation to their total volume and may have trouble keeping cool. This is one reason that these large animals tend to have sparse coverings of hair.

Summary

- Skin consists of two layers: the thin **epidermis** and under it the thicker **dermis.**
- The **Epidermis** is formed by the division of base cells that push those above them towards the surface where they die and are shed.
- **Keratin**, a protein, is deposited in the epidermal cells. It makes skin waterproof.
- Various skin structures formed in the epidermis are made of keratin. These include: claws, nails, hoofs, horn, hair and feathers.
- Various **Exocrine Glands** (with ducts) formed in the epidermis include sweat, sebaceous, and mammary glands.
- **Melanin** deposited in cells at the base of the epidermis protects deeper cells from the harmful effects of the sun.
- The **Dermis** is composed of loose connective tissue and is well supplied with blood.

- Beneath the dermis is insulating **adipose tissue**.
- Body Temperature is controlled by: sweat, hair erection, dilation and contraction of dermal capillaries and shivering.

Worksheet

Use the Skin Worksheet [2] to help you learn all about the skin.

Test Yourself

Now use this Skin Test Yourself to see how much you have learned and remember.

1. The two layers that form the skin are the a) and b)

a)epidermis

b)dermis

2. The special protein deposited in epidermal cells to make them waterproof is:

keratin

3. Many important skin structures are made of keratin. These include:

hair,nails,foot pads,feathers,scales on reptiles

4. Sweat, sebaceous and mammary glands all have ducts to the outside. These kind of glands are known as:

exocrine

5. What is the pigment deposited in skin cells that protects underlying skin layers from the harmful effects of the sun?

melanin

6. How does the skin help cool an animal down when it is active or in a hot environment?

Panting and secretion from sweat glands.

7. Name two mechanisms by means of which the skin helps prevent heat loss when an animal is in a cold environment.

a.shivering

b.contraction of blood vessels

Test Yourself Answers

Websites

- http://www.auburn.edu/academic/classes/zy/0301/Topic6/Topic6.html Comparative anatomy

Good on keratin skin structures - hairs, feathers, horns etc.

- http://www.olympusmicro.com/micd/galleries/brightfield/skinhairymammal.html Hairy mammal skin

All about hairy mammalian skin.

- http://www.earthlife.net/birds/feathers.html The wonder of bird feathers

Fantastic article on bird feathers with great pictures.

- http://en.wikipedia.org/wiki/Skin Wikipedia

Wikipedia on (human) skin. Good as usual, but more information than you need.

Glossary

- Link to Glossary [4]

References

[1] http://flickr.com/photos/alosojos/318955761/
[2] http://www.wikieducator.org/Skin_Worksheet

Anatomy and Physiology of Animals/The Skin/Test Yourself Answers

1. The two layers that form the skin are the: *epidermis and dermis*

2. The special protein deposited in epidermal cells to make them waterproof is *keratin*

3. Skin structures made of keratin include *scales, beaks, claws, nails, hoofs, hairs and feathers.*

4. Sweat, sebaceous and mammary glands are all *exocrine glands. Meaning they all have ducts through which they expel their products to the outside.*

5. The pigment deposited in skin cells that protects underlying skin layers from the harmful effects of the sun is *melanin.*

6. The skin helps cool an animal down when it is active or in a hot environment *by producing sweat and dilating the capillaries in the dermis*

7. The skin helps prevent heat loss when an animal is in a cold environment by:

   a) *contraction of the hair erector muscles to make the hairs stand up and trap an insulating layer of air.*

   b) *constriction of the capillaries in the dermis to reduce heat loss through the body surface.*

Anatomy and Physiology of Animals/The Skeleton

Objectives

After completing this section, you should know:

- the functions of the skeleton
- the basic structure of a vertebrae and the regions of the vertebral column
- the general structure of the skull
- the difference between 'true ribs' and 'floating ribs
- the main bones of the fore and hind limbs, and their girdles and be able to identify them in a live cat, dog, or rabbit

Fish, frogs, reptiles, birds and mammals are called **vertebrates**, a name that comes from the bony column of vertebrae (the spine) that supports the body and head. The rest of the skeleton of all these animals (except the fish) also has the same basic design with a skull that houses and protects the brain and sense organs and ribs that protect the heart and lungs and, in mammals, make breathing possible. Each of the four limbs is made to the same basic pattern. It is joined to the spine by means of a flat, broad bone called a **girdle** and consists of one long upper bone, two long lower bones, several smaller bones in the wrist or ankle and five digits (see diagrams 6.1 18,19 and 20).

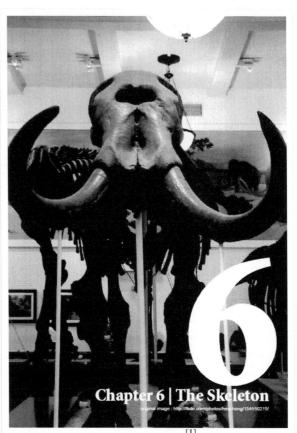

Chapter 6 | The Skeleton

original image by heschong [1] cc by

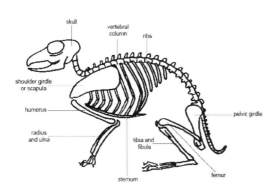

Diagram 6.1 - The mammalian skeleton

The Vertebral Column

The vertebral column consists of a series of bones called **vertebrae** linked together to form a flexible column with the skull at one end and the tail at the other. Each vertebra consists of a ring of bone with spines (spinous process) protruding dorsally from it. The spinal cord passes through the hole in the middle and muscles attach to the spines making movement of the body possible (see diagram 6.2).

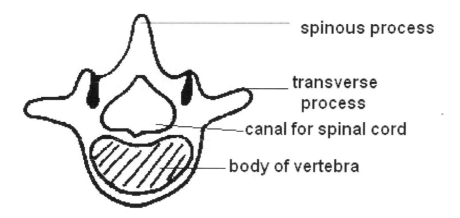

Diagram 6.2 - Cross section of a lumbar vertebre

The shape and size of the vertebrae of mammals vary from the neck to the tail. In the neck there are **cervical vertebrae** with the two top ones, the **atlas** and **axis**, being specialised to support the head and allow it to nod "Yes" and shake "No". **Thoracic vertebrae** in the chest region have special surfaces against which the ribs move during breathing. Grazing animals like cows and giraffes that have to support weighty heads on long necks have extra large spines on their cervical and thoracic vertebrae for muscles to attach to. **Lumbar vertebrae** in the loin region are usually large strong vertebrae with prominent spines for the attachment of the large muscles of the lower back. The **sacral vertebrae** are usually fused into one solid bone called the **sacrum** that sits within the **pelvic girdle**. Finally there are a variable number of small bones in the tail called the **coccygeal vertebrae** (see diagram 6.3).

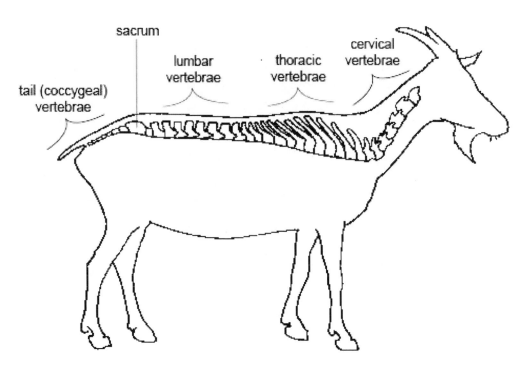

Diagram 6.3 - The regions of the vertebral column dik

The Skull

The skull of mammals consists of 30 separate bones that grow together during development to form a solid case protecting the brain and sense organs. The "box "enclosing and protecting the brain is called the **cranium** (see diagram 6.4). The bony wall of the cranium encloses the middle and inner ears, protects the organs of smell in the nasal cavity and the eyes in sockets known as **orbits**. The teeth are inserted into the upper and lower jaws (see Chapter 5 for more on teeth) The lower jaw is known as the **mandible**. It forms a joint with the skull moved by strong muscles that allow an animal to chew. At the front of the skull is the nasal cavity, separated from the mouth by a plate of bone called the **palate**. Behind the nasal cavity and connecting with it are the **sinuses**. These are air spaces in the bones of the skull which help keep the skull as light as possible. At the base of the cranium is the **foramen magnum**, translated as "big hole", through which the spinal cord passes. On either side of this are two small, smooth rounded knobs or **condyles** that **articulate** (move against) the first or Atlas vertebra.

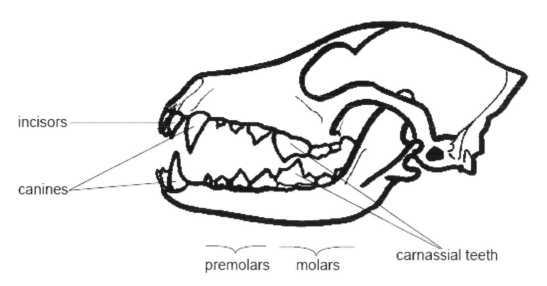

Diagram 6.4 - A dog's skull

The Rib

Paired ribs are attached to each thoracic vertebra against which they move in breathing. Each rib is attached ventrally either to the **sternum** or to the rib in front by cartilage to form the rib cage that protects the heart and lungs. In dogs one pair of ribs is not attached ventrally at all. They are called **floating ribs** (see diagram 6.5). Birds have a large expanded sternum called the **keel** to which the flight muscles (the 'breast" meat of a roast chicken) are attached.

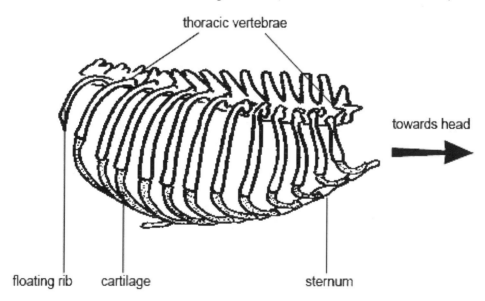

Diagram 6.5 - The rib

The Forelimb

The forelimb consists of: **Humerus, radius** and **ulna, carpals, metacarpals, digits** or **phalanges** (see diagram 6.6). The top of the humerus moves against (articulates with) the **scapula** at the shoulder joint. By changing the number, size and shape of the various bones, fore limbs have evolved to fit different ways of life. They have become wings for flying in birds and bats, flippers for swimming in whales, seals and porpoises, fast and efficient limbs for running in horses and arms and hands for holding and manipulating in primates (see diagram 6.8).

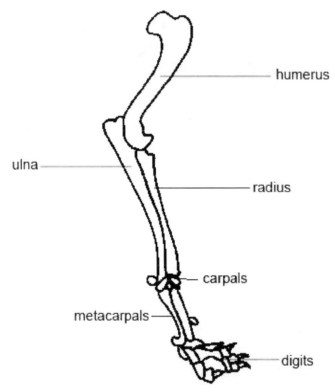

Diagram 6.6 - Forelimb of a dog

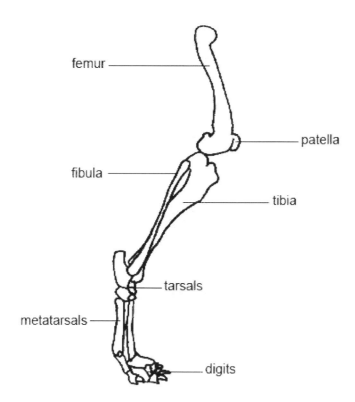

Diagram 6.7. Hindlimb of a dog

The Hind Limb

The hind limbs have a similar basic pattern to the forelimb. They consist of: **femur, tibia** and **fibula, tarsals, metatarsals, digits** or **phalanges** (see diagram 6.7). The top of the femur moves against (articulates with) the pelvis at the hip joint.

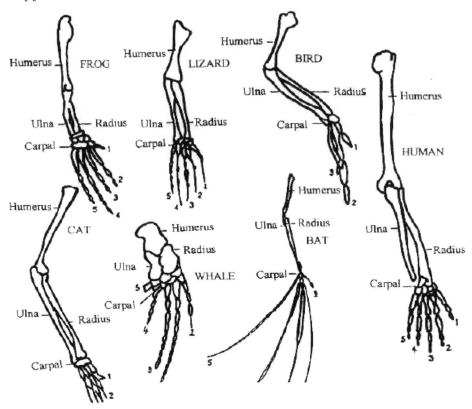

Diagram 6.8 - Various vertebrate limbs

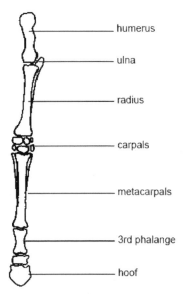

Diagram 6.9 - Forelimb of a horse

The **patella** or kneecap is embedded in a large tendon in front of the knee. It seems to smooth the movements of the knee. The legs of the horse are highly adapted to give it great galloping speed over long distances. The bones of the leg, wrist and foot are greatly elongated and the hooves are actually the tips of the third fingers and toes, the other digits having been lost or reduced (see diagram 6.9).

The Girdles

The girdles pass on the "push" produced by the limbs to the body. The shoulder girdle or **scapula** is a triangle of bone surrounded by the muscles of the back but not connected directly to the spine (see diagram 6.1). This arrangement helps it to cushion the body when landing after a leap and gives the forelimbs the flexibility to manipulate food or strike at prey. Animals that use their forelimbs for grasping, burrowing or climbing have a well-developed **clavicle** or collar bone. This connects the shoulder girdle to the sternum. Animals like sheep, horses and cows that use their forelimbs only for supporting the body and locomotion have no clavicle. The **pelvic girdle** or hipbone attaches the sacrum and the hind legs. It transmits the force of the leg-thrust in walking or jumping directly to the spine (see diagram 6.10).

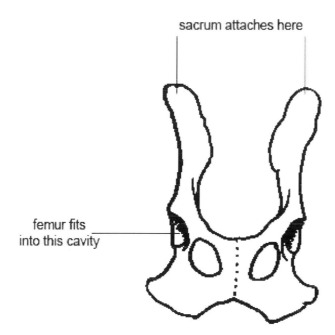

sacrum attaches here

femur fits into this cavity

Diagram 6.10 - The pelvic girdle

Categories Of Bones

People who study skeletons place the different bones of the skeleton into groups according to their shape or the way in which they develop. Thus we have **long bones** like the femur, radius and finger bones, **short bones** like the ones of the wrist and ankle, **irregular bones** like the vertebrae and **flat bones** like the shoulder blade and bones of the skull. Finally there are bones that develop in tissue separated from the main skeleton. These include **sesamoid bones** which include bones like the patella or kneecap that develop in tendons and **visceral bones** that develop in the soft tissue of the penis of the dog and the cow's heart.

Bird Skeletons

Although the skeleton of birds is made up of the same bones as that of mammals, many are highly adapted for flight. The most noticeable difference is that the bones of the forelimbs are elongated to act as wings. The large flight muscles make up as much as 1/5th of the body weight and are attached to an extension of the sternum called the **keel**. The vertebrae of the lower back are fused to provide the rigidity needed to produce flying movements. There are also many adaptations to reduce the weight of the skeleton. For instance birds have a beak rather than teeth and many of the bones are hollow (see diagram 6.11).

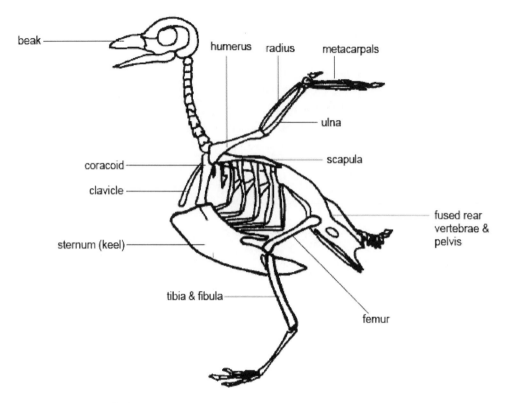

Diagram 6.11 - A bird's skeleton

The Structure Of Long Bones

A long bone consists of a central portion or **shaft** and two ends called **epiphyses** (see diagram 6.12). Long bones move against or articulate with other bones at joints and their ends have flattened surfaces and rounded protuberances (condyles) to make this possible. If you carefully examine a long bone you may also see raised or rough surfaces. This is where the muscles that move the bones are attached. You will also see holes (a hole is called a **foramen**) in the bone. Blood vessels and nerves pass into the bone through these. You may also be able to see a fine line at each end of the bone. This is called the **growth plate** or **epiphyseal line** and marks the place where increase in length of the bone occurred (see diagram 6.16).

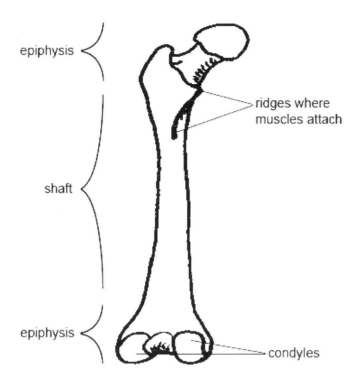

Diagram 6.12 - A femur

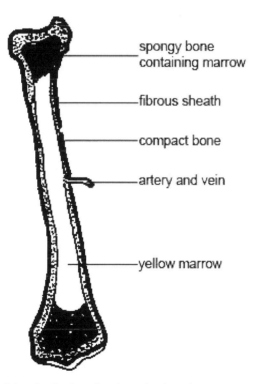

6.13 - A longitudinal section through a long bone

If you cut a long bone lengthways you will see it consists of a hollow cylinder (see diagram 6.13). The outer shell is covered by a tough fibrous sheath to which the tendons are attached. Under this is a layer of hard, dense **compact bone** (see below). This gives the bone its strength. The central cavity contains fatty **yellow marrow**, an important energy store for the body, and the ends are made from honeycomb-like bony material called **spongy bone** (see box below). Spongy bone contains **red marrow** where red blood cells are made.

Compact Bone

Compact bone is not the lifeless material it may appear at first glance. It is a living dynamic tissue with blood vessels, nerves and living cells that continually rebuild and reshape the bone structure as a result of the stresses, bends and breaks it experiences. Compact bone is composed of microscopic hollow cylinders that run parallel to each other along the length of the bone. Each of these cylinders is called a **Haversian system**. Blood vessels and nerves run along the central canal of each Haversian system. Each system consists of concentric rings of bone material (the **matrix**) with minute spaces in it that hold the bone cells. The hard matrix contains crystals of calcium phosphate, calcium carbonate and magnesium salts with collagen fibres that make the bone stronger and somewhat flexible. Tiny canals connect the cells with each other and their blood supply (see diagram 6.14).

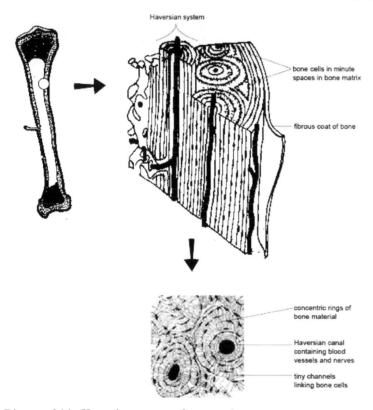

Diagram 6.14 - Haversian systems of compact bone

Spongy Bone

Spongy bone gives bones lightness with strength. It consists of an irregular lattice that looks just like an old fashioned loofah sponge (see diagram 6.15). It is found on the ends of long bones and makes up most of the bone tissue of the limb girdles, ribs, sternum, vertebrae and skull. The spaces contain red marrow, which is where red blood cells are made and stored.

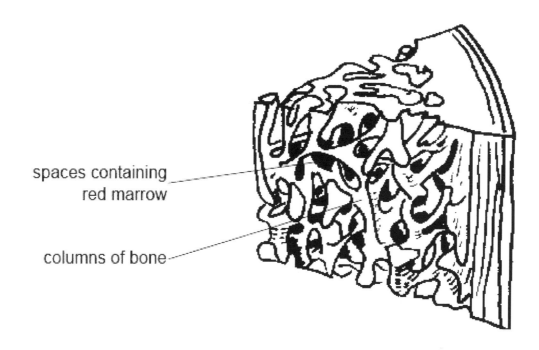

spaces containing
red marrow

columns of bone

Diagram 6.15 - Spongy bone

Bone Growth

The skeleton starts off in the foetus as either cartilage or fibrous connective tissue. Before birth and, sometimes for years after it, the cartilage is gradually replaced by bone. The long bones increase in length at the ends at an area known as the **epiphyseal plate** where new cartilage is laid down and then gradually converted to bone. When an animal is mature, bone growth ceases and the epiphyseal plate converts into a fine **epiphyseal line** (see diagram 6.16).

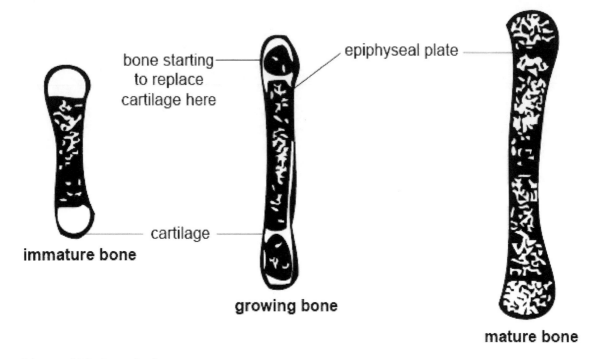

Diagram 6.16 - A growing bone

Broken Bones

A fracture or break dramatically demonstrates the dynamic nature of bone. Soon after the break occurs blood pours into the site and cartilage is deposited. This starts to connect the broken ends together. Later spongy bone replaces the cartilage, which is itself replaced by compact bone. Partial healing to the point where some weight can be put on the bone can take place in 6 weeks but complete healing may take 3-4 months.

Joints

Joints are the structures in the skeleton where 2 or more bones meet. There are several different types of joints. Some are **immovable** once the animal has reached maturity. Examples of these are those between the bones of the skull and the midline joint of the pelvic girdle. Some are **slightly moveable** like the joints between the vertebrae but most joints allow free movement and have a typical structure with a fluid filled cavity separating the articulating surfaces (surfaces that move against each other) of the two bones. This kind of joint is called a **synovial joint** (see diagram 6.17). The joint is held together by bundles of white fibrous tissue called **ligaments** and a fibrous **capsule** encloses the joint. The inner layers of this capsule secrete the **synovial fluid** that acts as a lubricant. The articulating surfaces of the bones are covered with **cartilage** that also reduces friction and some joints, e.g. the knee, have a pad of cartilage between the surfaces that articulate with each other.

The shape of the articulating bones in a joint and the arrangement of ligaments determine the kind of movement made by the joint. Some joints only allow a to and from **gliding movement** e.g. between the ankle and wrist bones; the joints at the elbow, knee and fingers are **hinge joints** and allow movement in two dimensions and the axis vertebra **pivots** on the atlas vertebra. **Ball and socket joints**, like those at the shoulder and hip, allow the greatest range of movement.

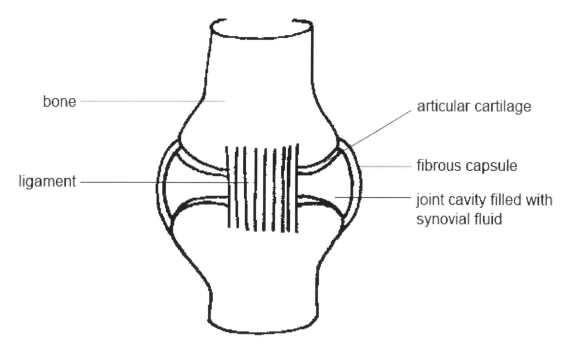

Diagram 6.17 - A synovial joint

Common Names Of Joints

Some joints in animals are given common names that tend to be confusing. For example:

1. The joint between the femur and the tibia on the hind leg is our knee but the **stifle** in animals.
2. Our ankle joint (between the tarsals and metatarsals) is the **hock** in animals
3. Our knuckle joint (between the metacarpals or metatarsals and the phalanges) is the **fetlock** in the horse.
4. The **"knee"** on the horse is equivalent to our wrist (ie on the front limb between the radius and metacarpals) see diagrams 6.6, 6.7, 6.8, 6.17 and 6.18.

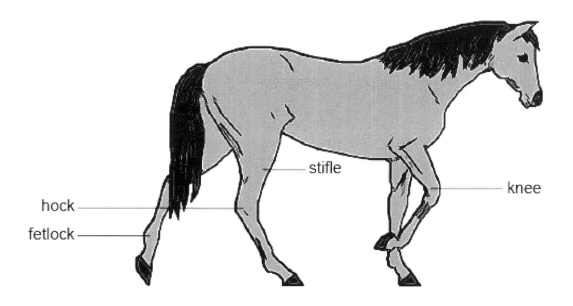

Diagram 6.18 - The names of common joints of a horse

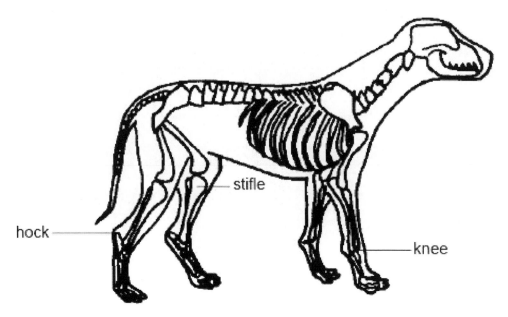

Diagarm 6.19 - The names of common joints of a dog

Locomotion

Different animals place different parts of the foot or forelimb on the ground when walking or running.

Humans and bears put the whole surface of the foot on the ground when they walk. This is known as **plantigrade locomotion**. Dogs and cats walk on their toes (**digitigrade locomotion**) while horses and pigs walk on their "toenails" or hoofs. This is called **unguligrade locomotion** (see diagram 6.20).

1. **Plantigrade locomotion** (on the "palms of the hand) as in humans and bears
2. **Digitigrade locomotion** (on the "fingers") as in cats and dogs
3. **Unguligrade locomotion** (on the "fingernails") as in horses

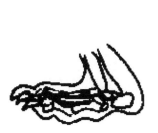 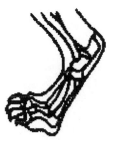 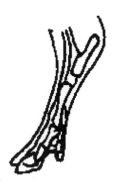

Diagram 6.20 - Locomotion

Summary

- The skeleton maintains the shape of the body, protects internal organs and makes locomotion possible.
- The **vertebrae** support the body and protect the spinal cord. They consist of: **cervical vertebrae** in the neck, **thoracic vertebrae** in the chest region which articulate with the ribs, **lumbar vertebrae** in the loin region, **sacral vertebrae** fused to the pelvis to form the sacrum and **tail** or **coccygeal vertebrae**.
- The **skull** protects the brain and sense organs. The **cranium** forms a solid box enclosing the brain. The **mandible** forms the jaw.
- The forelimb consists of the **humerus, radius, ulna, carpals, metacarpals** and **phalanges**. It moves against or **articulates** with the **scapula** at the shoulder joint.
- The hindlimb consists of the **femur, patella, tibia, fibula, tarsals, metatarsals** and **digits**. It moves against or articulates with the **pelvis** at the hip joint.
- Bones articulate against each other at **joints**.
- **Compact bone** in the shaft of long bones gives them their strength. **Spongy bone** at the ends reduces weight. Bone growth occurs at the **growth plate**.

Worksheet

Use the Skeleton Worksheet [2] to learn the main parts of the skeleton.

Test Yourself

1. Name the bones which move against (articulate with)...

    a) the humerus:

    b) the thoracic vertebrae:

    c) the pelvis:

2. Name the bones in the forelimb:

3. Where is the patella found?

4. Where are the following joints located?

    a) The stifle joint:

    b) The elbow joint:

    c) The hock joint:

    d) The hip joint:

5. Attach the following labels to the diagram of the long bone shown below.

    a) compact bone

    b) spongy bone

    c) growth plate

    d) fibrous sheath

    e) red marrow

    f) blood vessel

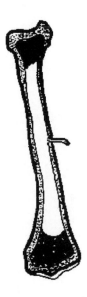

6. Attach the following labels to the diagram of a joint shown below

     a) bone

     b) articular cartilage

     c) joint cavity

     d) capsule

     e) ligament

     f) synovial fluid.

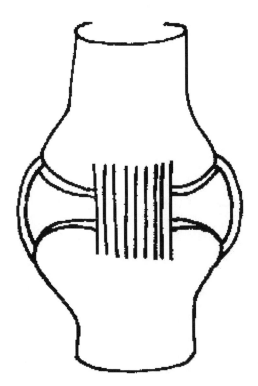

Test Yourself Answers

Websites

- http://www.infovisual.info/02/056_en.html Bird skeleton

A good diagram of the bird skeleton.

- http://www.earthlife.net/mammals/skeleton.html Earth life

A great introduction to the mammalian skeleton. A little above the level required but it has so much interesting information it's worth reading it.

- http://www.klbschool.org.uk/interactive/science/skeleton.htm The human skeleton

Test yourself on the names of the bones of the (human) skeleton.

- http://www.shockfamily.net/skeleton/JOINTS.HTML The joints

Quite a good article on the different kinds of joints with diagrams.

- http://en.wikipedia.org/wiki/Bone Wikipedia

Wikipedia is disappointing where the skeleton is concerned. Most articles stick entirely to the human skeleton or have far too much detail. However this one on compact and spongy bone and the growth of bone is quite good although still much above the level required.

Glossary

- Link to Glossary [4]

References

[1] http://flickr.com/photos/heschong/154550215/
[2] http://www.wikieducator.org/Skeleton_Worksheet

Anatomy and Physiology of Animals/The Skeleton/Test Yourself Answers

1. Name the bones which move against (articulate with)...

    a) the humerus: *moves against the scapula, radius and ulna.*

    b) the thoracic vertebrae: *move against adjacent cranial and caudal vertebrae & the ribs*

    c) the pelvis: *moves against the femur and the sacrum*

2. Name the bones in the forelimb:

    From the scapula are the *humerus, radius, ulna, carpals, metacarpals and digits.*

3. Where is the patella found?

    The patella is the knee cap. It is found in the hind limb at the knee joint.

4. Where are the following joints located?

    a) The stifle joint: *between the femur and the tibia on the hind limb.*

    b) The elbow joint: *between the humerus, radius and ulna on the forelimb.*

    c) The hock joint: *between the tarsals and metatarsals on the hind limb.*

    d) The hip joint: *between the pelvis and the femur.*

5. Attach the following labels to the diagram of the long bone shown below.

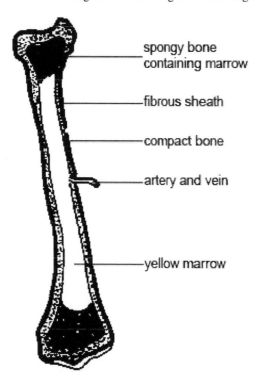

spongy bone
containing marrow

fibrous sheath

compact bone

artery and vein

yellow marrow

6. Attach the following labels to the diagram of a joint shown below.

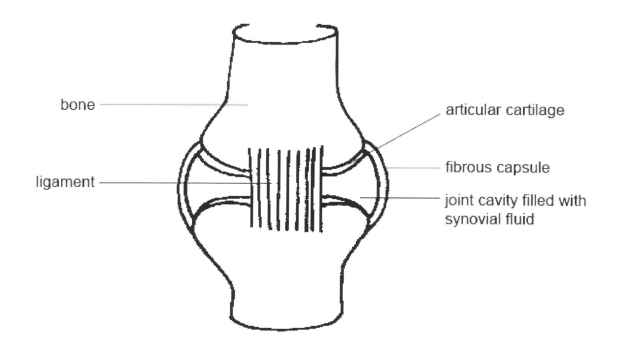

bone

ligament

articular cartilage

fibrous capsule

joint cavity filled with synovial fluid

Anatomy and Physiology of Animals/Muscles

Objectives

After completing this section, you should know:

- the structure of smooth, cardiac and skeletal muscle and where they are found
- what the insertion and origin of a muscle is
- what flexion and extension of a muscle means
- that muscles usually operate as antagonistic pairs
- what tendons attach muscles to bones

Muscles

Muscles make up the bulk of an animal's body and account for about half its weight. The meat on the chop or roast is muscle and is composed mainly of protein. The cells that make up muscle tissue are elongated and able to contract to a half or even a third of their length when at rest. There are three different kinds of muscle; smooth, cardiac and skeletal muscle.

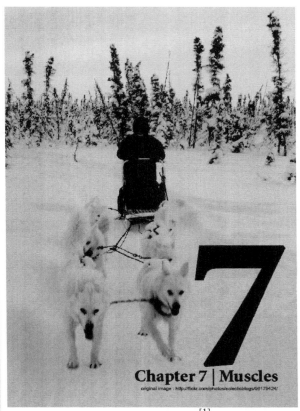

Chapter 7 | Muscles

original image : http://flickr.com/photos/eclecticblogs/90179424/

original image by eclecticblogs [1] cc by

Smooth muscle

Smooth or Involuntary muscle carries out the unconscious routine tasks of the body such as moving food down the digestive system, keeping the eyes in focus and adjusting the diameter of blood vessels. The individual cells are spindle-shaped, being fatter in the middle and tapering off towards the ends with a nucleus in the centre of the cell. They are usually found in sheets and are stimulated by the non-conscious or autonomic nervous system as well as by hormones (see Chapter 3).

Cardiac muscle

Cardiac muscle is only found in the wall of the heart. It is composed of branching fibres that form a three-dimensional network. When examined under the microscope, a central nucleus and faint stripes or striations can be seen in the cells. Cardiac muscle cells contract spontaneously and rhythmically without outside stimulation but the pacemaker coordinates the heart beat. Nerves and hormones modify this rhythm (see Chapter 3).

Skeletal muscle

Skeletal muscle is the muscle that is attached to and moves the skeleton, and is under voluntary control. It is composed of elongated cells or fibres lying parallel to each other. Each cell is unusual in that it has several nuclei and when examined under the microscope appears striped or striated. This appearance gives the muscle its names of striped or striated muscle. Each cell of striated muscle contains hundreds, or even thousands, of microscopic fibres each one with its own striped appearance. The stripes are formed by two different sorts of protein that slide over each other making the cell contract (see diagram 7.1).

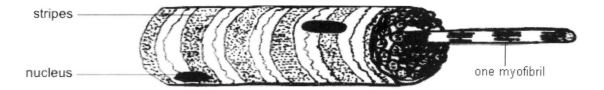

Diagram 7.1 - A striped muscle cell

Muscle contraction

Muscle contraction requires energy and muscle cells have numerous mitochondria. However, only about 15% of the energy released by the mitochondria is used to fuel muscle contraction. The rest is released as heat. This is why exercise increases body temperature and makes animals sweat or pant to rid themselves of this heat.

What we refer to as a muscle is made up of groups of muscle fibres surrounded by connective tissue. The connective tissue sheaths join together at the ends of the muscle to form tough white bands of fibre called **tendons**. These attach the muscles to the bones. Tendons are similar in structure to the **ligaments** that attach bones together across a joint (see diagrams 7.2a and b).

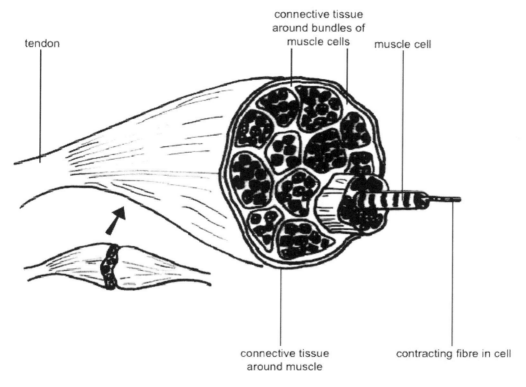

Diagram 7.2 a and b - The structure of a muscle

Remember:

Tendons Tie muscles to bones

              and

Ligaments Link bones at joints

Structure of a muscle

A single muscle is fat in the middle and tapers towards the ends. The middle part, which gets fatter when the muscle contracts, is called the **belly** of the muscle. If you contract your biceps muscle in your upper arm you may feel it getting fatter in the middle. You may also notice that the biceps is attached at its top end to bones in your shoulder while at the bottom it is attached to bones in your lower arm. Notice that the bones at only one end move when you contract the biceps. This end of the muscle is called the **insertion**. The other end of the muscle, the **origin**, is attached to the bone that moves the least (see diagram 35).

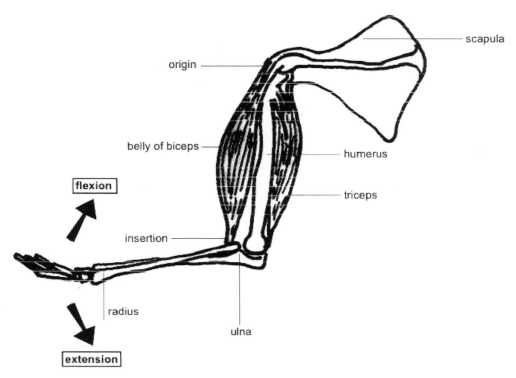

Diagram 7.3 - Antagonistic muscles, flexion and extension

Antagonistic muscles

Skeletal muscles usually work in pairs. When one contracts the other relaxes and vice versa. Pairs of muscles that work like this are called **antagonistic muscles**. For example the muscles in the upper forearm are the biceps and triceps (see diagram 7.3). Together they bend the elbow. When the biceps contracts (and the triceps relaxes) the lower forearm is raised and the angle of the joint is reduced. This kind of movement is called **flexion**. When the triceps is contracted (and the biceps relaxes), the angle of the elbow increases. The term for this movement is **extension**.

When you or animals contract skeletal muscle it is a voluntary action. For example, you make a conscious decision to walk across the room, raise the spoon to your mouth or smile. There is however, another way in which contraction of muscles attached to the skeleton happens that is not under voluntary control. This is during a **reflex action**, such as jerking your hand away from the hot stove you have touched by accident. This is called a **reflex arc** and will be described in detail in chapter 14-15.

Summary

- There are three different kinds of muscle tissue: **smooth muscle** in the walls of the gut and blood vessels; **cardiac muscle** in the heart and **skeletal muscle** attached to the skeleton.

- **Tendons** attach skeletal muscles to the skeleton.

- **Ligaments** link bones together at a joint.

- Skeletal muscles work in pairs known as **antagonistic pairs.** As one contracts the other in the pair relaxes.

- **Flexion** is the movement that reduces the angle of a joint. **Extension** increases the angle of a joint.

Test Yourself

1. What kind of muscle tissue:

   a) moves bones:

   b) makes the heart pump blood:

   c) pushes food along the intestine:

   d) makes your mouth form a smile:

   e) makes the hair stand up when cold:

   f) makes the diaphragm contract for breathing in:

2. What structure connects a muscle to a bone?

3. What is the insertion of a muscle?

4. Which muscle is antagonistic to the biceps?

5. When you flex your knee what movement are you making?

6. When you extend your ankle joint what happens?

Test Yourself Answers

Website

- http://health.howstuffworks.com/muscle.htm How muscles work

Description of the three types of muscles and how skeletal muscles work.

Glossary

- Link to Glossary [4]

References

[1] http://flickr.com/photos/eclecticblogs/96179424/

Anatomy and Physiology of Animals/Muscles/Test Yourself Answers

1. What kind of muscle tissue:

   a) *Skeletal muscle* moves bones.

   b) *Cardiac muscle* makes the heart pump blood.

   c) *Smooth muscle* pushes food along the intestine.

   d) Smiling is a voluntary action (usually!) so *skeletal muscle* is involved.

   e) You cannot control "Goosebumps" so the muscles involved are *smooth muscles*.

   f) Although breathing seems to be involuntary most of the time it is possible to control it voluntarily so the diaphragm (the main breathing muscle) is a *skeletal muscle*.

2. What structure connects a muscle to a bone?

   A *tendon* connects a muscle to a bone.

3. What is the insertion of a muscle? *The insertion of a muscle is the end attached to the bone that moves most when the muscle contracts.*

4. Which muscle is antagonistic to the biceps?

   The triceps is the muscle that forms the other half of the antagonistic pair with the biceps.

5. When you flex your knee what movement are you making?

   When you flex your knee you bend your knee.

6. When you extend your ankle joint what happens?

   When you extend your ankle joint you point your toes.

Anatomy and Physiology of Animals/Cardiovascular System

This chapter on the Cardiovascular system is divided into 3 sections. These are:

1. Blood
2. The Heart
3. Blood circulation

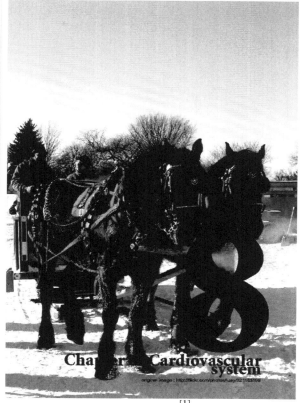

original image by tuey [1] cc by

References

[1] http://flickr.com/photos/tuey/321163599

Anatomy and Physiology of Animals/Cardiovascular System/Blood

Objectives

After completing this section, you should know:

- the main functions of blood
- what the term haematocrit or packed cell volume (PCV) means
- what is in blood
- what plasma is and what is in it
- the appearance and function of red blood cells (RBCs)
- the appearance and function of white blood cells particularly granulocytes, lymphocytes and
    monocytes
- the function of platelets and fibrinogen in blood clotting
- how oxygen and carbon dioxide are transported in the blood
- the names of some anticoagulants and their function in the body and in the vet clinic

Blood

Blood is a unique fluid containing cells that is pumped by the heart around the body of animals in a system of pipes known as the **circulatory system**. It carries oxygen and nutrients to the cells of the body and removes waste products like carbon dioxide from them. Blood is also important for keeping conditions in the body constant, in other words for maintaining **homeostasis**. It helps keep the acidity or pH stable and helps maintain a constant temperature in the body. Blood also has an important role in defending the body against disease.

A simple way to find out what is in blood is to remove a small amount from an animal and place it in a tube with a substance that prevents it from clotting (an **anticoagulant**). If you leave the tube to stand for a few hours you will find that it settles out into two layers. The top layer consists of a light yellow fluid, the **plasma**, and the bottom layer consists of **red blood cells** (RBCs). If you look very carefully you can also see a thin beige-coloured layer in between these two layers. This consists of the **white blood cells** (WBCs) (see diagram 8.1).

The above procedure is usually done more rapidly by placing the blood sample in a centrifuge for a few minutes. This machine acts like a super spin drier rotating about 10,000 times a minute and packing the heavier particles (red blood cells) at the bottom of the tube. The sample that results is called the **packed cell volume (P.C.V.)** or haematocrit. It is a very useful measurement of the concentration of red blood cells in the blood. For most animals the packed cell volume is in the range 30-45%. If it is lower than this it means that the concentration of red blood cells is low and the animal is **anaemic**. If the reading is above this range it may mean the animal is **dehydrated.** Animals that live at high altitudes also have high P.C.V.s to compensate for the low oxygen concentration there.

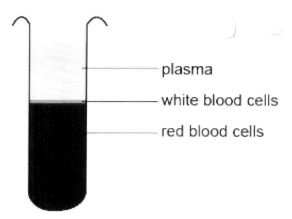

Diagram 8.1 - Packed cell volume of blood

Plasma

Plasma consists of water (91%) in which many substances are dissolved. These dissolved substances include:

- salts (or electrolytes)
- proteins
- nutrients
- waste products
- dissolved gases (mainly carbon dioxide)
- and other chemicals like hormones

Salts in Plasma

Salts in the plasma are in the form of **ions** or **electrolytes** which include sodium, potassium, calcium, chloride, phosphate and bicarbonate. Plasma transports these ions to where they are needed e.g. calcium required by the bones, they also help keep the osmotic pressure and acid-base balance (pH) of the blood within the required levels.

Blood Proteins

The proteins in the blood plasma are large molecules with important functions. Some contribute to the **osmotic pressure** (see chapter 3) and the viscosity (thickness) of the blood, and so help keep the blood volume and pressure stable. Others act as **antibodies** that attack bacteria and viruses, and yet others are important in blood **clotting**. Nutrients that are absorbed from the gut and transported to the cells in the plasma include amino acids, glucose, fatty acids and vitamins. Waste products include urea from the breakdown of proteins.

Red Blood Cells

Red blood cells are also known as RBCs or **erythrocytes**. They are what make blood red. When you look at a blood smear through a microscope, as you will in one of the practical classes, you will see that RBCs are by far the most common cells in the blood. (In fact there are about 5 million per millilitre). If you focus on an individual RBC you will see that they are shaped like discs or doughnuts with a thin central portion surrounded by a fatter margin. This shape has all sorts of advantages, one being that enables the cells to fold up and pass along the narrowest blood capillaries (See diagram 8.2).

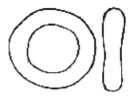

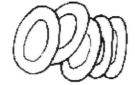

Front and side
view of a red blood cell

Red blood cell
cut in half

Red blood cells as they
appear in a blood clot

Diagram 8.2 - Red blood cells or erythrocytes

The mature RBCs of mammals have neither nucleus nor other organelles and can be thought of as sacks of **haemoglobin**. Haemoglobin is a red coloured protein containing iron, which joins with oxygen so the blood can transport it to body cells. RBCs are made continuously in the bone marrow and live about 120 days. They are then destroyed in the liver and spleen and the molecules they are made from recycled to make new RBCs. Anaemia results if the rate at which RBCs are **destroyed** exceeds the rate at which RBC'c are **produced**.

Note that if you happen to look at bird's, reptiles, frogs or fishes blood down the microscope you will see that these vertebrates all have RBCs with a central nucleus.

White Blood Cells

White blood cells or **leucocytes** are far less numerous than red blood cells. In fact there is only about one white cell for every 1000 red blood cells. Rather than being white, they are actually colourless as they contain no haemoglobin although unlike RBCs they do have a nucleus. If you make a blood smear and look at it under the microscope it is difficult to see the white blood cells at all. To make them visible you need to stain them with special dyes or stains. There are a variety of stains that can be used, but most dye the nucleus a dark purple or pink colour. The stains may also show up the granules present in the cytoplasm of some white blood cells. White blood cells are divided into two major groups depending on the shape of the nucleus and whether or not there are granules in the cytoplasm.

1.**Granulocytes** or **polymorphonuclear leucocytes** ("polymorphs" or "polys") have granules in the cytoplasm and a purple lobed nucleus (see diagram 8.3). The most common (**neutrophils**) can squeeze out of capillaries and are involved in engulfing and destroying foreign invaders like bacteria (see diagram 8.4). Some (**eosinophils**) combat allergies and increase in numbers during parasitic worm infections. Others (**basophils**) produce **heparin** that prevents the blood from clotting.

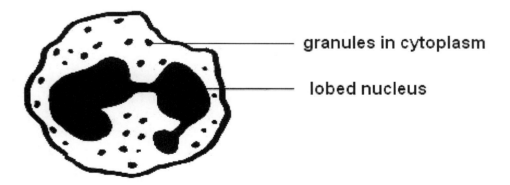

granules in cytoplasm

lobed nucleus

Diagram 8.3 - A granulocyte

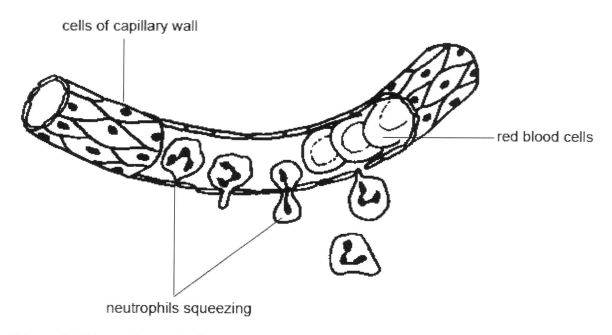

Diagram 8.4 - Neutrophils escaping from a capillary

2. **Agranulocytes** or **monomorphonuclear leucocytes** have a large unlobed nucleus and no granules in the cytoplasm. There are two types of agranulocytes. The most numerous are **lymphocytes** that are concerned with immune responses. The second type is the **monocyte** that is the largest blood cell and is involved in engulfing bacteria etc. by phagocytosis (see diagram 8.5).

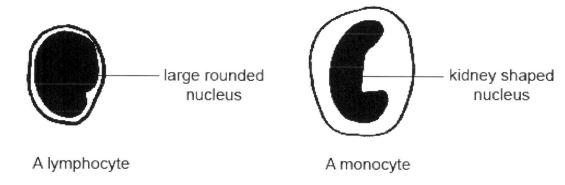

Diagram 8.5 - Agranular leucocytes

Platelets

As well as red and white blood cells, the blood also contains small irregular shaped fragments of cells known as platelets. They are involved in the clotting of the blood (see later).

Transport Of Oxygen

The purpose of the haemoglobin in red blood cells is to carry oxygen from the lungs to the tissues. In fact it allows the blood to carry about 25 times more oxygen than it would be able to without any haemoglobin.

When oxygen concentrations are high, as in the blood capillaries in the lungs, haemoglobin combines with oxygen to form a compound called **oxyhaemoglobin**. This compound is bright red and makes the **oxygenated blood** that spurts from a damaged artery its characteristic bright red colour. When the blood reaches the tissues where the oxygen concentrations are low, the oxygen separates from the haemoglobin and diffuses into the tissues. The haemoglobin in most veins has given up its oxygen and the blood is called **deoxygenated blood**. It is a purple-red colour.

Carbon Monoxide Poisoning

Carbon monoxide is a colourless, odourless gas found in car exhaust fumes and tobacco smoke. It combines with haemoglobin just like oxygen but does not let go. This means the haemoglobin molecules are not available to carry oxygen to the tissues and the animal or human suffocates. Carbon monoxide poisoning is often fatal but can be treated by giving the patient pure oxygen that slowly replaces the carbon monoxide.

Transport Of Carbon Dioxide

Carbon dioxide is a waste gas produced by cells. It diffuses into the blood capillaries where it is carried to the lungs in the blood. Most is carried in the plasma as **bicarbonate ions** but a small amount is dissolved directly in the plasma and some combines with haemoglobin.

Transport Of Other Substances

The blood carries water to the cells and organs as well as soluble food substances (sugars, amino acids, fatty acids and vitamins) and hormones dissolved in the plasma. These are delivered to the cells via the **tissue fluid** (see later in this chapter) that surrounds them. Blood also picks up the waste products like carbon dioxide and urea from the cells and is important in distributing the heat produced in the liver and muscles all over the body.

Blood Clotting

The mechanism that causes the blood to clot is easily seen when you or your animals are injured. However, minor injuries occur all the time in areas that experience wear and tear like the intestine, the lungs and the skin. Without the clotting mechanism, animals would quickly bleed to death from minor injury and internal **haemorrhage.** This is what happens in animals and people with clotting disorders like haemophilia, as well as animals that are poisoned with rat poisons like warfarin.

Platelets are important in blood clotting. When blood vessels are damaged, substances released cause the blood platelets to disintegrate. This stimulates a complex chain of reactions, which causes the protein **fibrinogen** to be converted to **fibrin**. Fibrin forms a dense fibrous network over the wound preventing the escape of further blood. **Calcium** and **vitamin K** are essential for the clotting process and any deficiency of these may also lead to clotting problems.

Serum And Plasma

When blood clots it separates into the clot that contains most of the cells and platelets leaving behind a straw coloured fluid. This fluid is called **serum**. It looks just like plasma and is similar in composition except for one big difference. It doesn't contain fibrinogen, the protein that forms the clot.

Anticoagulants

Anticoagulants are substances that interfere with the clotting process. When blood is collected for transfusion or testing it is often important to prevent it clotting and there are a number of different anticoagulants you can use for this. Tubes containing the different anticoagulants are coded with different colours for easy recognition.

1. **Heparin** (colour code - green) is a natural anticoagulant produced by the white blood cells but it is also used routinely in the laboratory with samples to be tested for heavy metals like lead.
2. **EDTA** (colour code – lavender) is used for routine blood counts.
3. **Fluoroxylate** (colour code – grey) is used for biochemical tests for glucose.
4. **Citrate** (colour code – light blue) is used for the storage of large quantities of blood, such as used in transfusions.

Haemolysis

Haemolysis is the breakdown of the plasma membrane of red blood cells to release the haemoglobin. We have already met this process when discussing osmosis, for haemolysis often occurs when red blood cells are placed in a hypotonic solution and water flows in through the semi permeable plasma membrane to swell and eventually burst the cell. It is therefore important when collecting blood from an animal to make sure there is no water in the syringe or tube. Too much movement due to shaking the tube or sucking up the blood too vigorously can also break down the plasma membrane and cause haemolysis.

Blood Groups

If you have given blood recently you may know your blood group. It may be blood group O, A or B or even AB, the rarest group. Blood groups are the result of different molecules called antigens on the outside of red blood cells. These cause antibodies to be formed that attack viruses and bacteria. Knowledge of a person's blood group is important when giving transfusions because if blood of another incompatible blood group is given to a patient the red blood cells stick together and block the blood vessels and may lead to death.

Blood groups also exist in many animals. There are three blood groups in cats and great care has to be taken that the groups are compatible when transfusing exotic breeds. The situation is slightly different in dogs. They have a number of blood groups but there is usually no problem with the first blood transfusion a dog receives. However, this first transfusion sensitises the immune system so that a problem may arise with the second and subsequent transfusions.

Haemolysis can occur in the living animal when it is exposed to various poisons and toxins. This may happen when, for example, it eats a poisonous plant, is bitten by a snake or infected with bacteria that destroy red blood cells (haemolytic bacteria).

Blood Volume

Blood accounts for between 6-10% of the body weight of animals, varying with the species and the stage of life. Animals can not tolerate losses of greater than 3% of the total volume when the condition known as **shock** occurs.

Summary | Blood

- The main functions of blood are transport of oxygen, food, waste products etc., the maintenance of homeostasis and defending the body from disease.
- Blood consists of fluid, plasma, in which red and white blood cells are suspended. The blood cells typically make up 30-45% of the blood volume.
- Plasma consists of water containing dissolved substances like proteins, nutrients and carbon dioxide.
- Red Blood Cells contain **haemoglobin** to transport **oxygen**.
- **White Blood Cells** defend the body from invasion. There are 2 kinds:
- **Granular white cells** include **neutrophils, basophils** and **eosinophils**. Neutrophils which destroy bacteria are the most numerous. Eosinophils are involved with allergies and parasitic infections.
- **Non-granular white cells** include **lymphocytes** that produce antibodies to attach bacteria and viruses and **monocytes** that engulf and destroy bacteria and viruses.
- **Platelets** are involved in blood clotting.

Worksheet

The exercises in the Blood Worksheet [1] will help you learn how to identify the different types of blood cell and what their functions are.

Test Yourself

1. The liquid part of blood is known as:

2. There are two main types of cells in blood. They are:

    a)

    b)

3. The most numerous cells in blood are:

4. The main function of the red blood cells is:

5. How would you tell a white cell from a red cell when looking at them through a microscope? (Give at least 2 differences)

6. How does the blood help fight invasion by bacteria and viruses?

7. What would happen to blood if there were no platelets?

Test Yourself Answers

Websites

- http://www.getbodysmart.com/ap/circulatory/heart/menu/heart.html Get Body Smart

Shows constituents of blood including RBCs, white cells, platelets and plasma. Even shows how to make a blood smear and identify the white cells on it as well as make and read a haematocrit. Some parts are a little too advanced.

- Wikipedia has good information of red and white blood cells.
  - http://en.wikipedia.org/wiki/Red_blood_cell Red blood cells
  - http://en.wikipedia.org/wiki/White_blood_cell White blood cells

Glossary

- Link to Glossary [4]

References

[1] http://www.wikieducator.org/Blood_Worksheet

Anatomy and Physiology of Animals/Cardiovascular System/Blood/Test Yourself Answers

1. The liquid part of blood is known as *plasma*

2. There are two main types of cells in blood. They are:

   a) *red blood cells*

   b) *white blood cells*.

3. The most numerous cells in blood are *red blood cells*

4. The main function of the red blood cells is *to transport oxygen.*

5. How would you tell a white cell from a red cell when looking at them through a microscope? (Give at least 2 differences)

   You would tell a white cell from a red cell when looking at them through a microscope by the red (pink) colour and no nucleus of red blood cells compared to the white cells which have a colourless cytoplasm and a purple stained nucleus.

6. How does the blood help fight invasion by bacteria and viruses?

   White cells in the blood help fight invasion by bacteria and viruses by engulfing them (neutrophils and monocytes) or producing chemicals (antibodies) that kill them (lymphocytes).

7. What would happen to blood if there were no platelets?

   If there were no platelets in the blood it would not clot to stop bleeding.

Anatomy and Physiology of Animals/Cardiovascular System/The Heart

Objectives | The Heart

After completing this section, you should know:

- where the heart is located in the body
- the structure of the heart
- the structure and function of the heart valves and their role in producing the heart sounds
- the stages of the heart beat and the route the blood takes through the heart
- that the coronary arteries supply the heart muscle

The Heart

The heart is the pump that pushes the blood around the body in the blood vessels of the **circulatory** system. **In fishes the blood only passes through the heart once on its way to the gills and then** round the rest of the body. However, in mammals and birds that have lungs, the blood passes through the heart twice: once on its way to the lungs where it picks up oxygen and then through the heart again to be pumped all over the body. The heart is therefore two separate pumps, side by side (see diagram 8.6).

The heart is situated in the thorax between the lungs and is protected by the rib cage. In some animals it is displaced slightly to the left-hand side. A tough membrane called the **pericardium** covers it. There is a narrow space between the pericardium and the heart that is filled with a liquid that acts as a lubricant.

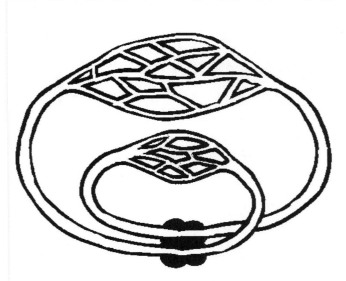

Diagram 8.6: The double closed circulation of a mammal

The heart of mammals is a hollow bag made of cardiac muscle (see chapter 4). The cavity inside the heart is divided into 4 chambers. The chambers on the right side are completely separate from the chambers on the left side. The two upper chambers are thin walled, and are called the **atria** (or auricles). The two lower chambers are thick walled and are called the **ventricles** (see diagrams 8.7 and 8.8).

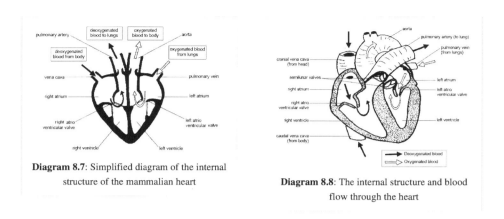

Diagram 8.7: Simplified diagram of the internal structure of the mammalian heart

Diagram 8.8: The internal structure and blood flow through the heart

The Heart

Blood flows through the heart in a one way system. The right atrium receives deoxygenated blood from the body via the largest vein in the body called the **vena cava**. The contraction of the atrium pumps the blood into the right ventricle and then into the lungs via the **pulmonary artery**. The blood is oxygenated in the lungs and then returns to the heart and enters the left atrium via the **pulmonary vein**. The contraction of the left atrium pumps the blood into the left ventricle, which then pumps it to the body via the **aorta** (see diagrams 8.7 and 8.8). The wall of the left ventricle is usually much thicker than that of the right ventricle because it has to pump the blood to the end of the digits and tip of the tail while the right ventricle only has to pump the blood to the nearby lungs.

Valves

Valves are flaps of tissue that stop blood flowing backwards and so control the direction of blood flow in the heart. There are two kinds of valves in the heart. The first kind is the massive valves between the atria and the ventricles, the **atrio-ventricular valves**, (AV valves) that prevent blood in the ventricles from flowing back into the atria. The flaps of these valves are attached to the walls of the ventricles by tendons. These make them look somewhat like parachutes (see diagram 8.9).

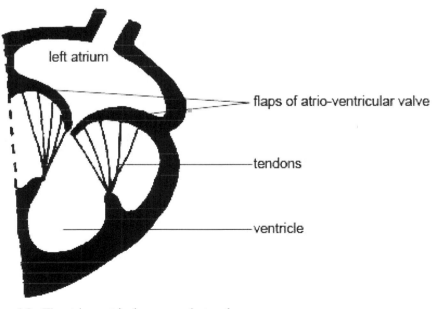

Diagram 8.9 - The atrio-ventricular or parachute valves

The second kind of valve is pocket shaped flaps of tissue called the **semilunar** (half moon) **valves** (see diagram 8). They are called the **pulmonary and aortic valves** and found at the back of the pulmonary artery and aorta respectively.

The Heartbeat

The heartbeat consists of alternating contractions and relaxations of the heart. It you listen to the heart with a stethoscope you hear the sounds often described as "**lubb-dupp**".

There are four stages to each heartbeat:

1. Each atrium relaxes so that blood can enter. Blood flows from the body via the vena cava into the :right atrium. At the same time, blood flows from the lungs via the pulmonary vein into the left :atrium (see diagram 8.10a).
2. The atrio-ventricular valves open and both ventricles relax. The atria contract and blood flows from the right atrium into the right ventricle and from the left atrium into the left ventricle (see diagram 8.10b).
3. The ventricles contract and the atrio-ventricular valves snap shut to stop blood flowing back into the atria. This is the first sound ("lubb") of the heartbeat that can be heard with a stethoscope (see diagram 8.10c).
4. The semi-lunar valves open and blood is pumped out of the right ventricle to the lungs. At the same time, blood is pumped out of the left ventricle into the aorta and so to the rest of the body. When the ventricles stop contracting the semi-lunar valves snap shut to stop blood flowing backwards.

This is the second sound ("dupp") of the heartbeat. Blood flows into the atria again as they relax and the cycle is repeated.

When a valve is damaged and fails to close completely some blood may flow backwards after each heartbeat. A trained veterinarian hears this with a stethoscope as a "**heart murmur**".

The period of the heart beat when the ventricles are contracting and sending a wave of blood down the pulmonary artery and aorta is called **systole**. The period when the ventricles are relaxing is called **diastole**.

Cardiac Muscle

The walls of the heart consist of cardiac muscle, a special kind of muscle only found in the heart. The cells of cardiac muscle form a branching network of separating and rejoining fibres which allows nerve impulses to travel through the tissue (see Chapter 7). Heart muscle needs lots of energy to function so it is well supplied with mitochondria and requires a good supply of oxygen. This is provided by the coronary arteries (see below).

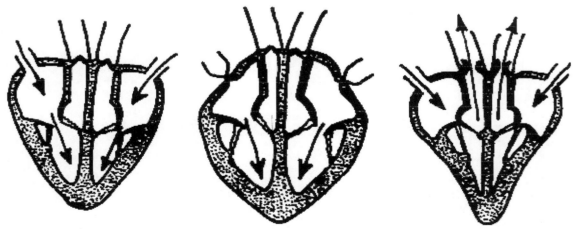

Diagram 8.10 a) First stage of heartbeat b) Second stage of heartbeat c) Third stage of heartbeat

Control Of The Heartbeat

The cardiac muscle of the walls of the heart contracts of its own accord. This can be demonstrated by the rather macabre experiment in which a small portion of heart muscle is removed and placed in a solution that is similar to blood. The tissue will continue to contract and relax for a time. In the normal functioning heart the **pacemaker** acts rather like the conductor of an orchestra and superimposes a unified beat upon the heart as a whole. The pacemaker is situated in the wall of the right atrium. The rate at which the heart beats is modified by a part of the brain called the **medulla oblongata** (see Chapter 14) and by the hormone adrenalin (see Chapter 16) which speeds up the heartbeat.

The Coronary Vessels

Although oxygenated blood passes through some of the chambers of the heart it can not supply the muscle of the heart walls with the oxygen and nutrients it needs. Special arteries called the **coronary arteries** do this. These two arteries arise from the aorta and branch through the heart to deliver oxygen and nutrients to the cardiac muscles and collect carbon dioxide and wastes. Coronary veins return the blood to right hand side of the heart. Some of these vessels can be seen on the outside surface of the heart (see diagram 8.11). Sometimes fatty deposits on the inside wall of the coronary artery block the blood flow to the heart muscle. If the obstruction is severe enough to damage the heart muscle due to inadequate blood supply a "heart attack" can result.

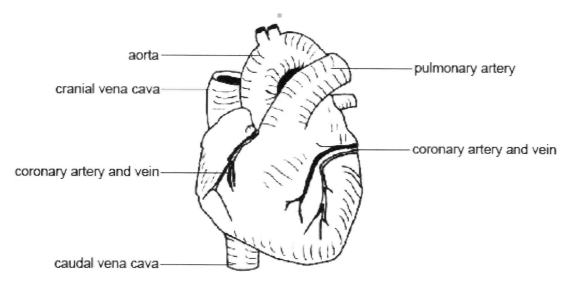

Diagram 8.11 - The heart showing coronary vessels

Summary

- The heart is situated in the thorax between the lungs
- The heart is a hollow bag made of **cardiac muscle**. It is divided into four chambers (right and left atria and right and left ventricles).
- Valves stop blood flowing backwards. The right and left **atrio-ventricular valves** prevent blood in the ventricles from flowing back into the atria. The **semilunar valves** at the entrance of the pulmonary artery and aorta prevent blood flowing back into the ventricles. The closing of the valves produces the heart sounds heard with a stethoscope.
- There are 4 stages to the heart beat. 1. blood flows into the right and left atria. 2. The atria contract and blood flows into the ventricles. 3. The ventricles contract and the closing of the atrio-ventricular valves produces the first heart sound. 4. Blood flows to the lungs and body and when the ventricles stop contracting the closing of the

semilunar valves produces the second heart sound.

- The **coronary arteries** supply the heart muscle with oxygenated blood.

Worksheet

Use the Heart Worksheet [1] to help you learn the different parts of the heart, the role of the heart valves and how the heart beat pushes the blood through the heart.

Test Yourself

1. Via what vessel does blood enter the heart from the body?
2. Blood passing through the right atrioventricular valve passes into which chamber of the heart?
3. What is the function of the pulmonary valve?
4. Does the pulmonary artery carry deoxygenated or oxygenated blood?
5. The walls of the heart are made of what tissue?
6. Does the aorta carry deoxygenated or oxygenated blood?

Test Yourself Answers

Websites on the Heart

- http://www.guidant.com/condition/heart/heart_bloodflow.shtml Blood flow through heart

An animation of blood flow through the heart with step-by-step annotated breakdown. Also an animation putting heartbeat, valve operation and blood flow all together.

- http://www.getbodysmart.com/ap/circulatory/heart/menu/heart.html Get Body Smart

Great animation showing parts of heart plus constituents of blood including RBCs, white cells, platelets and plasma. Even shows how to make a blood smear and identify the white cells on it as well as make and read a haematocrit. Some parts are a little too advanced.

- http://www.bishopstopford.com/faculties/science/arthur/Heart%20drag&drop.swf Heart animation

Drag and drop animation of the human heart. Great for revision but note the terms bicuspid and tricuspid valves are used. These are equivalent to the left and right atrio-ventricular valves in animals.

- http://www.guidant.com/condition/heart/heart_valves.shtml Heart beat

A good animation of the heartbeat showing the valves opening and closing with appropriate heart sounds. Plus a good diagram showing the difference between the atrio-ventricular and semilunar valves.

- http://www.nucleusinc.com/animation2.php Human heart animation

A great animation where you use the mouse to point to parts of the heart and a voice over tells you what part it is. Just note this is of the human heart so the terms superior and inferior vena cava are used instead of caudal and cranial as for an animal.

- http://en.wikipedia.org/wiki/Heart The heart

Again Wikipedia is a wonderful resource, although remember, most of the material is on the human system.

Glossary

- Link to Glossary [4]

References

[1] http://www.wikieducator.org/Heart_Worksheet

Anatomy and Physiology of Animals/Cardiovascular System/The Heart/Test Yourself Answers

1. Via what vessel does blood enter the heart from the body?

   Blood enter the heart from the body via the cranial and caudal vena cavae.

2. Blood passing through the right atrioventricular valve passes into which chamber of the heart?

   Into the right ventricle.

3. What is the function of the pulmonary valve?

   The pulmonary valve prevents backflow of blood from the pulmonary artery into the right ventricle.

4. Does the pulmonary artery carry deoxygenated or oxygenated blood?

   The pulmonary artery carries deoxygenated blood.

5. The walls of the heart are made of what tissue?

   The walls of the heart are made of cardiac muscle.

6. Does the aorta carry deoxygenated or oxygenated blood?

   The aorta carries oxygenated blood.

Anatomy and Physiology of Animals/Cardiovascular System/Blood circulation

Objectives | Blood Circulation

After completing this section, you should know:

- that the circulatory system is double consisting of pulmonary and systemic circuits with the blood :passing through the heart twice;
- the differences in the structure and function of arteries, capillaries and veins;
- how the pulse is produced and where it can be felt;
- what tissue fluid and lymph are and how they are formed;
- the names of the main arteries and veins.

Blood Circulation

The circulatory system is the continuous system of tubes through which the blood is pumped around the body. It supplies the tissues with their requirements and removes waste products. In mammals and birds the blood circulates through two separate systems - the first from the heart to the lungs and back to the heart again (the pulmonary circulation) and the second from the heart to the head and body and back again (the systemic circulation) (see diagram 8.12).

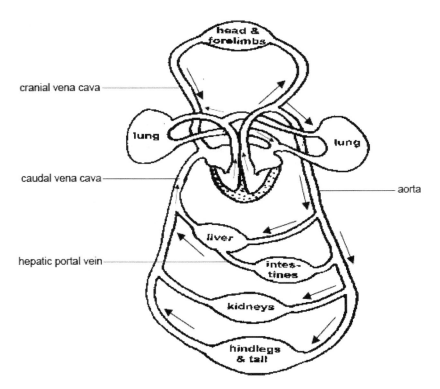

Diagram 8.12 - The mammalian circulatory system

The tubes through which the blood flows are the **arteries, capillaries** and **veins**. The heart pumps blood into arteries that carry it away from the heart. The arteries divide into very thin vessels called capillaries that form a network between the cells of the body. The capillaries then join up again to make veins that return the blood to the heart.

Arteries

Arteries carry blood away from the heart. They have thick elastic walls that stretch and can withstand the surges of high pressure blood caused by the heartbeat (the pulse, see later). The arteries divide into smaller vessels called **arterioles**. The hole down the centre of the artery is called the **lumen**. There are three layers of tissue in the walls of an artery. It is lined with squamous epithelial cells. The middle layer is the thickest layer. It made of elastic fibres and smooth muscle to make it stretchy. The outer fibrous layer protects the artery (see diagram 8.13). The **pulse** is only felt in arteries.

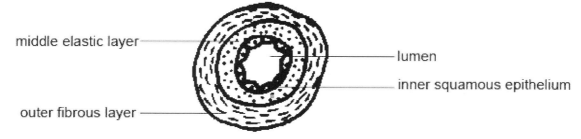

middle elastic layer
lumen
inner squamous epithelium
outer fibrous layer

Diagram 8.13 - Cross section of an artery

The Pulse

The pulse is the spurt of high pressure blood that passes along the aorta and arteries when the left ventricle contracts. As the pulse of blood passes along an artery the elastic walls stretch. When the pulse has passed the walls contract and this helps push the blood along. The pulse is easily felt at certain places where an artery passes near the surface of the body. It is strongest near the heart and becomes weaker as it travels away from the heart. The pulse disappears altogether in the capillaries.

Capillaries

Arterioles divide repeatedly to form a network penetrating between the cells of all tissues of the body. These small vessels are called capillaries. The walls are only one cell thick and some capillaries are so narrow that red blood cells have to fold up to pass through them. Capillaries form networks in tissues called capillary beds. The capillary networks in capillary beds are so dense that no living cell is far from its supply of oxygen and food (see diagram 8.14).

Note: All arteries carry oxygenated blood except for the pulmonary artery that carries deoxygenated blood to the lungs.

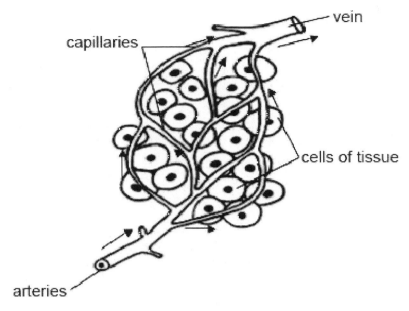

capillaries

vein

cells of tissue

arteries

Diagram 8.14 - A capillary bed

The Formation Of Tissue Fluid And Lymph

The thin walls of capillaries allow water, some white blood cells and many dissolved substances to diffuse through them. These form a clear fluid called **tissue fluid** (or **extracellular fluid** or **interstitial fluid**) that surrounds the cells of the tissues. The tissue fluid allows oxygen and nutrients to pass from the blood to the cells and carbon dioxide and other waste products to be removed from the tissues (see diagram 8.15).

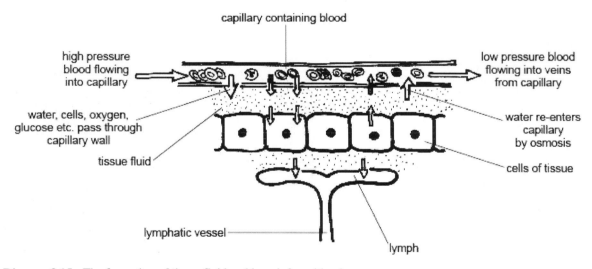

capillary containing blood

high pressure blood flowing into capillary

low pressure blood flowing into veins from capillary

water, cells, oxygen, glucose etc. pass through capillary wall

water re-enters capillary by osmosis

tissue fluid

cells of tissue

lymphatic vessel

lymph

Diagram 8.15 - The formation of tissue fluid and lymph from blood

Some tissue fluid finds its way back into the capillaries and some of it flows into the blind-ended lymphatic vessels that form a network in the tissues. Once the tissue fluid has entered the lymphatics it is called **lymph** although its composition remains the same. The lymph vessels have walls that are even thinner than the capillaries. This means that molecules and particles that are larger than those that can pass into the blood stream e.g. cancer cells and bacteria can enter the lymphatic system. These are then filtered out as the lymph passes through lymph nodes. (See chapter 10 for more information on the lymphatic system).

Veins

Capillaries unite to form larger vessels called **venules** that join to form veins. Veins return blood to the heart and since blood that flows in veins has already passed through the fine capillaries, it flows slowly with no pulse and at low pressure. For this reason veins have thinner walls than arteries although there have the same three layers in them as arteries (see diagram 8.16). As there is no pulse in veins, the blood is squeezed along them by the contraction of the skeletal muscles that lay alongside them.

Veins also have **valves** in them that prevent blood flowing backwards (see diagram 8.17a and b).

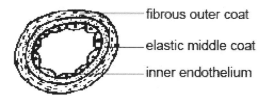

Diagram 8.16 - Cross section of a vein

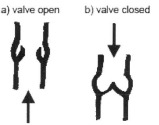

Diagram 8.17 a) and b) Valves in a vein

Note: Most veins carry deoxygenated blood. The pulmonary vein that carries oxygenated blood from the lungs to the left atrium of the heart is an exception.

Regulation Of Blood Flow

The flow of blood along arteries, arterioles and capillaries is not constant but can be controlled depending upon the requirements of the body. For example more blood is directed to the skeletal muscles, brain or digestive system when they are active. Regulation of the blood flow to the arterioles of the skin is also important in controlling body temperature. The size of the vessels is adjusted by the contraction or relaxation of smooth muscle fibres in their walls.

Oedema And Fluid Loss

Oedema is the swelling of the tissues due to the accumulation of tissue fluid. This may occur because the tissue fluid is prevented from returning to the bloodstream and accumulates in the tissues. This may be caused by physical inactivity (e.g. long car or plane trips in humans) or because of imbalances in the proteins in the blood. This is what causes the "pot-belly" of the malnourished child or worm-infested puppy.

Loss of body fluid can be caused not only by drinking insufficient liquid but also through diarrhea and vomiting or sudden loss of blood due to **haemorrhage.** The effect is to reduce the volume of the blood which decreases the blood pressure. This could be dangerous because the supply of adequate blood to the brain depends upon maintaining the blood pressure at a constant level.

To compensate for the loss of fluid various mechanisms come into play. First of all the blood vessels contract in order to try and maintain the pressure. Then, since the loss of fluid tends to make the blood more concentrated and increases its osmotic pressure, fluid is drawn into the blood from the tissues by osmosis.

The Spleen

The spleen is situated near the stomach. It has a rich blood supply and acts as a reservoir of red blood cells. When there is a sudden loss of blood, as happens when a haemorrhage occurs, the spleen contracts to release large numbers of red blood cells into the circulation. The spleen also destroys old red cells and makes new lymphocytes but it is not an essential organ because its removal in adult life seems to cause few problems. In the foetus, the spleen makes both red and white cells.

Important Blood Vessels Of The Systemic (Body) Circulation

Blood is pumped out into the body via the main artery, the **aorta**. This takes the blood to the head, the limbs and all the body organs. After passing through a network of fine capillaries, the blood is returned to the heart in the largest vein, the **vena cava** (see diagrams 8.8, 8.12, 8.18 and 8.19).

Arteries and veins to and from many organs often run alongside each other and have the same name e.g. the **renal artery and vein** serve the kidney, the **femoral artery and vein** serve the hind limbs and the **subclavian artery and vein** serve the forelimbs. However, blood to the head passes along the **carotid artery** and returns to the cranial vena cava via the **jugular vein**.

One variation on this arrangement is found in the blood vessels that serve the digestive tract. A variety of arteries take blood from the aorta to the intestines but blood from the intestines is carried by the **hepatic portal vein** to the liver where the digested food can be processed (see diagram 8.12). This vessel is unlike others in that it transports blood from one organ to another rather than to or from the heart like arteries or veins.

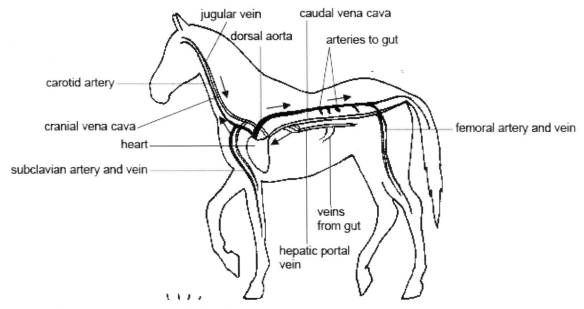

Diagram 8.18 - The main arteries and veins of the horse

Blood Pressure

The blood pressure is the pressure of the blood against the walls of the main arteries. The pressure is highest as the pulse produced by the contraction of the left ventricle passes along the artery. This is known as the **systolic pressure**. Pressure is much lower between pulses. This is known as the **diastolic pressure**. Blood pressure is measured in millimetres of mercury. A blood pressure that is higher than expected is known as **hypertension** while a pressure lower than expected is known as **hypotension.**

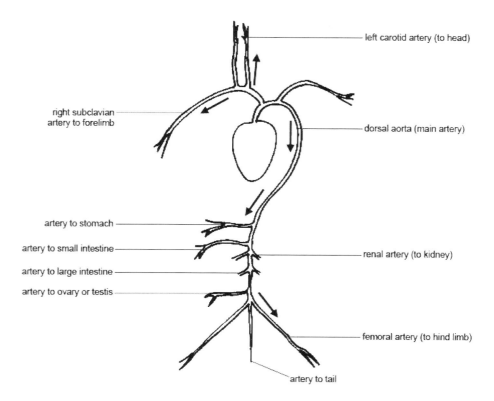

Diagram 8.19 - The main arteries of the body

Summary

- The circulatory system is double with the blood passing through the heart twice.
- **Arteries** carry blood away from the heart. They have thick elastic walls that stretch and can withstand the high pressure of the pulse.
- **Capillaries** are small, thin walled vessels that form a network between the cells of the tissues.
- **Veins** return low pressure blood to the heart. They have thinner walls than arteries.
- The **pulse** is the spurt of high pressure blood that passes along the arteries when the left ventricle contracts. It can be felt where arteries pass close to the body surface.
- **Tissue fluid** is the clear fluid that leaks from the capillaries and surrounds the cells of the tissues. **Lymph** forms when tissue fluid enters lymphatics.
- Important blood vessels include the vena cava, aorta, pulmonary artery, carotid artery, jugular vein, renal artery and vein and hepatic portal vessel.

Worksheet

This Circulatory System Worksheet [1] will help you learn the main vessels of the circulatory system, the difference between arteries and veins, and what happens in a capillary bed.

Test Yourself

1. Give 2 other differences between arteries and veins

    1.

    2.

2. What is systole?

3. Circle the correct answer below.

    Blood flows by this route through the blood vessels of the body.

    a) heart I veins I capillaries I arteries I heart

    b) heart I arteries I capillaries I veins I heart

    c) heart I veins I arteries I capillaries I heart

    d) heart I capillaries I arteries I veins I heart

4. Name the vessel that carries blood:

    from the heart to the main organs of the body:

    from the aorta to the brain:

    from the aorta to the kidneys:

    from the intestines to the liver:

    from the aorta to the heart muscle:

    from the aorta to the heart muscle:

Test Yourself Answers

Websites

- Wikipedia has good information on the circulatory system, although remember, most of the material is on the human system.
  - http://en.wikipedia.org/wiki/Circulatory_system Circulatory System
  - http://en.wikipedia.org/wiki/Blood_vessel Arteries and veins

Glossary

- Link to Glossary [4]

References

[1] http://www.wikieducator.org/Circulatory_System_Worksheet

Anatomy and Physiology of Animals/Cardiovascular System/Blood circulation/Test Yourself Answers

1. Does the pulse pass down arteries or veins?

   The pulse passes down arteries.

2. Give 2 other differences between arteries and veins. *Arteries have thicker walls than veins. Veins have valves to prevent backflow of blood.*

3. What is systole?

   Systole is the period when the ventricles are contracting and sending a wave of high-pressure blood (the pulse) along the aorta and arteries of the body.

4. Circle the correct answer below. Blood flows by this route through the blood vessels of the body.

   b) *heart | arteries | capillaries | veins | heart*

11. Name the vessel that carries blood:

    from the heart to the main organs of the body:*aorta*

    from the aorta to the brain: *carotid artery*

    from the aorta to the kidneys: *renal artery*

    from the intestines to the liver: *hepatic portal vessel*

    from the aorta to the heart muscle: *coronary artery*

Anatomy and Physiology of Animals/Respiratory System

Objectives

After completing this section, you should know:

- why animals need energy and how they make it in cells
- why animals require oxygen and need to get rid of carbon dioxide
- what the term gas exchange means
- the structure of alveoli and how oxygen and carbon dioxide pass across their walls
- how oxygen and carbon dioxide are carried in the blood
- the route air takes in the respiratory system (i.e. the nose, pharynx, larynx, trachea, bronchus, bronchioles, alveoli)
- the movements of the ribs and diaphragm to bring about inspiration
- what tidal volume, minute volume and vital capacity are
- how the rate of breathing is controlled and how this helps regulate the acid-base balance of the blood

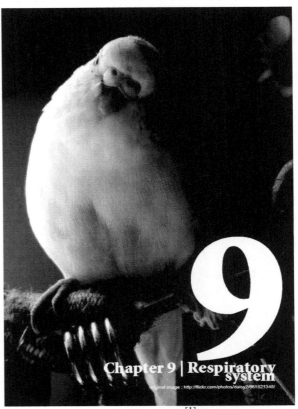

original image by Zofia P [1] cc by

Overview

Animals require a supply of energy to survive. This energy is needed to build large molecules like proteins and glycogen, make the structures in cells, move chemicals through membranes and around cells, contract muscles, transmit nerve impulses and keep the body warm. Animals get their energy from the large molecules that they eat as food. Glucose is often the energy source but it may also come from other carbohydrates, as well as fats and protein. The energy is made by the biochemical process known as **cellular respiration** that takes place in the **mitochondria** inside every living cell.

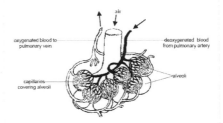

Diagram 9.1: Alveoli with blood supply

The overall reaction can be summarised by the word equation given below.

Charbohydrate Food (glucose) + Oxygen = Carbon Dioxide + Water + energy

As you can see from this equation, the cells need to be supplied with **oxygen** and **glucose** and the waste product, **carbon dioxide**, which is poisonous to cells, needs to be removed. The way the digestive system provides the glucose for cellular respiration will be described in Chapter 5, but here we are only concerned with the two gases, oxygen and carbon dioxide, that are involved in cellular respiration. These gases are carried in the blood to and from the tissues where they are required or produced.

Oxygen enters the body from the air (or water in fish)and carbon dioxide is usually eliminated from the same part of the body. This process is called **gas exchange**. In fish gas exchange occurs in the gills, in land dwelling vertebrates lungs are the gas exchange organs and frogs use gills when they are tadpoles and lungs, the mouth and the skin when adults.

Mammals (and birds) are active and have relatively high body temperatures so they require large amounts of oxygen to provide sufficient energy through cellular respiration. In order to take in enough oxygen and release all the carbon dioxide produced they need a very large surface area over which gas exchange can take place. The many minute air sacs or **alveoli** of the lungs provide this. When you look at these under the microscope they appear rather like bunches of grapes covered with a dense network of fine capillaries (see diagram 9.1). A thin layer of water covers the inner surface of each alveolus. There is only a very small distance -just 2 layers of thin cells - between the air in the alveoli and the blood in the capillaries. The gases pass across this gap by **diffusion**.

Diffusion And Transport Of Oxygen

The air in the alveoli is rich in oxygen while the blood in the capillaries around the alveoli is deoxygenated. This is because the haemoglobin in the red blood cells has released all the oxygen it has been carrying to the cells of the body. Oxygen diffuses from high concentration to low concentration. It therefore crosses the narrow barrier between the alveoli and the capillaries to enter the blood and combine with the haemoglobin in the red blood cells to form **oxyhaemoglobin**.

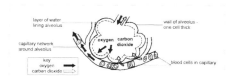

Diagram 9.2: Cross section of an alveolus

The narrow diameter of the capillaries around the alveoli means that the blood flow is slowed down and that the red cells are squeezed against the capillary walls. Both of these factors help the oxygen diffuse into the blood (see diagram 9.2).

When the blood reaches the capillaries of the tissues the oxygen splits from the haemoglobin molecule. It then diffuses into the tissue fluid and then into the cells.

Diffusion And Transport Of Carbon Dioxide

Blood entering the lung capillaries is full of carbon dioxide that it has collected from the tissues. Most of the carbon dioxide is dissolved in the plasma either in the form of **sodium bicarbonate** or **carbonic acid**. A little is transported by the red blood cells. As the blood enters the lungs the carbon dioxide gas diffuses through the capillary and alveoli walls into the water film and then into the alveoli. Finally it is removed from the lungs during breathing out (see diagram 9.2). (See chapter 8 for more information about how oxygen and carbon dioxide are carried in the blood).

The Air Passages

When air is breathed in it passes from the nose to the alveoli of the lungs down a series of tubes (see diagram 9.3). After entering the nose the air passes through the **nasal cavity**, which is lined with a moist membrane that adds warmth and moisture to the air as it passes. The air then flows through the **pharynx** or throat, a passage that carries both food and air, to the **larynx** where the voice-box is located. Here the passages for food and air separate again. Food must pass into the oesophagus and the air into the windpipe or **trachea**. To prevent food entering this, a small flap of tissue called the **epiglottis** closes the opening during swallowing (see chapter 11). A reflex that inhibits breathing during swallowing also (usually) prevents choking on food.

The trachea is the tube that ducts the air down the throat. Incomplete rings of cartilage in its walls help keep it open even when the neck is bent and head turned. The fact that acrobats and people that tie themselves in knots doing yoga still keep breathing during the most contorted manoeuvres shows how effective this arrangement is. The air passage now divides into the two **bronchi** that take the air to the right and left lungs before dividing into smaller and smaller **bronchioles** that spread throughout the lungs to carry air to the alveoli. Smooth muscles in the walls of the bronchi and bronchioles adjust the diameter of the air passages.

The tissue lining the respiratory passages produces **mucus** and is covered with minute hairs or **cilia.** Any dust that is breathed into the respiratory system immediately gets entangled in the mucous and the cilia move it towards the mouth or nose where it can be coughed up or blown out.

The Lungs And The Pleural Cavities

The lungs fill most of the chest or **thoracic cavity**, which is completely separated from the abdominal cavity by the **diaphragm**. The lungs and the spaces in which they lie (called the **pleural cavities**) are covered with membranes called the **pleura**. There is a thin film of fluid between the two membranes. This lubricates them as they move over each other during breathing movements.

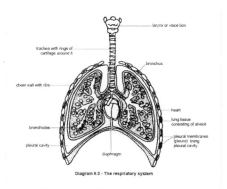

Diagram 9.3: The respiratory system

Collapsed Lungs

The pleural cavities are completely airtight with no connection with the outside and if they are punctured by accident (a broken rib will often do this), air rushes in and the lung collapses. Separating the two lungs is a region of tissue that contains the oesophagus, trachea, aorta, vena cava and lymph nodes. This is called the **mediastinum**. In humans and sheep it separates the cavity completely so that puncturing one pleural cavity leads to the collapse of only one lung. In dogs, however, this separation is incomplete so a puncture results in a complete collapse of both lungs.

Breathing

The process of breathing moves air in and out of the lungs. Sometimes this process is called **respiration** but it is important not to confuse it with the chemical process, **cellular respiration**, that takes place in the mitochondria of cells. Breathing is brought about by the movement of the diaphragm and the ribs.

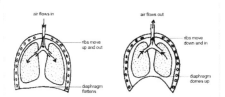

Diagram 9.4a: Inspiration; **Diagram 9.4b**: Expiration

Inspiration

The diaphragm is a thin sheet of muscle that completely separates the abdominal and thoracic cavities. When at rest it domes up into the thoracic cavity but during breathing in or **inspiration** it flattens. At the same time special muscles in the chest wall move the ribs forwards and outwards. These movements of both the diaphragm and the ribs cause the volume of the thorax to increase. Because the pleural cavities are airtight, the lungs expand to fill this increased space and air is drawn down the trachea into the lungs (see diagram 9.4a).

Expiration

Expiration or breathing out consists of the opposite movements. The ribs move down and in and the diaphragm resumes its domed shape so the air is expelled (see diagram 9.4b). Expiration is usually passive and no energy is required (unless you are blowing up a balloon).

Lung Volumes

As you sit here reading this just pay attention to your breathing. Notice that your in and out breaths are really quite small and gentle (unless you have just rushed here from somewhere else!). Only a small amount of the total volume that your lungs hold is breathed in and out with each breath. This kind of gentle "at rest" breathing is called **tidal breathing** and the volume breathed in or out (they should be the same) is the **tidal volume** (see diagram 9.5). Sometimes people want to measure the volume of air inspired or expired during a minute of this normal breathing. This is called the **minute volume**. It could be

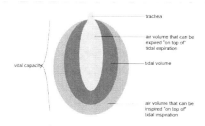

Diagram 9.5: Lung volumes

estimated by measuring the volume of one tidal breath and then multiplying that by the number of breaths in a minute. Of course it is possible to take a deep breath and breathe in as far as you can and then expire as far as possible. The volume of the air expired when a maximum expiration follows a maximum inspiration is called the **vital capacity** (see diagram 9.5).

Composition Of Air

The air animals breathe in consists of 21% oxygen and 0.04% carbon dioxide. Expelled air consists of 16% oxygen and 4.4% carbon dioxide. This means that the lungs remove only a quarter of the oxygen contained in the air. This is why it is possible to give someone (or an animal) artificial respiration by blowing expired air into their mouth.

Breathing is usually an unconscious activity that takes place whether you are awake or asleep, although, humans at least, can also control it consciously. Two regions in the hindbrain called the **medulla oblongata** and **pons** control the rate of breathing. These are called **respiratory centres**. They respond to the concentration of carbon dioxide in the blood. When this concentration rises during a bout of activity, for example, nerve impulses are automatically sent to the diaphragm and rib muscles that increase the rate and the depth of breathing. Increasing the rate of breathing also increases the amount of oxygen in the blood to meet the needs of this increased activity.

The Acidity Of The Blood And Breathing

The degree of acidity of the blood (the **acid-base balance**) is critical for normal functioning of cells and the body as a whole. For example, blood that is too acidic or alkaline can seriously affect nerve function causing a coma, muscle spasms, convulsions and even death. Carbon dioxide carried in the blood makes the blood acidic and the higher the concentration of carbon dioxide the more acidic it is. This is obviously dangerous so there are various mechanisms in the body that bring the acid-base balance back within the normal range. Breathing is one of these homeostatic mechanisms. By increasing the rate of breathing the animal increases the amount of dissolved carbon dioxide that is expelled from the blood. This reduces the acidity of the blood.

Breathing In Birds

Birds have a unique respiratory system that enables them to respire at the very high rates necessary for flight. The lungs are relatively solid structures that do not change shape and size in the same way as mammalian lungs do. Tubes run through them and connect with a series of air sacs situated in the thoracic and abdominal body cavities and some of the bones. Movements of the ribs and breastbone or sternum expand and compress these air sacs so they act rather like bellows and pump air through the lungs. The evolution of this extremely efficient system of breathing has enabled birds to migrate vast distances and fly at altitudes higher than the summit of Everest.

Summary

- Animals need to breathe to supply the cells with oxygen and remove the waste product **carbon dioxide**.
- The lungs are situated in the **pleural cavities** of the **thorax**.
- **Gas exchange** occurs in the **alveoli** of the lungs that provide a large surface area. Here oxygen diffuses from the alveoli into the red blood cells in the capillaries that surround the alveoli. Carbon dioxide, at high concentration in the blood, diffuses into the alveoli to be breathed out.
- **Inspiration** occurs when muscle contraction causes the ribs to move up and out and the diaphragm to flatten. These movements increase the volume of the pleural cavity and draw air down the respiratory system into the lungs.
- The air enters the nasal cavity and passes to the **pharynx** and **larynx** where the **epiglottis** closes the opening to the lungs during swallowing. the air passes down the trachea kept open by rings of cartilage to the **bronchi** and **bronchioles** and then to the alveoli.
- **Expiration** is a passive process requiring no energy as it relies on the relaxation of the muscles and recoil of the elastic tissue of the lungs.
- The rate of breathing is determined by the concentration of carbon dioxide in the blood. As carbon dioxide makes blood acidic, the rate of breathing helps control the **acid/base balance** of the blood.
- The cells lining the respiratory passages produce mucus which traps dust particles, which are wafted into the nose by cilia.

Worksheet

Work through the Respiratory System Worksheet [2] to learn the main structures of the respiratory system and how they contribute to inspiration and gas exchange.

Test Yourself

Then use the Test Yourself below to see how much you remember and understand.

1. What is meant by the phrase "gas exchange"?

2. Where does gas exchange take place?

3. What is the process by which oxygen moves from the alveoli into the blood?

4. Why does this process occur?

5. How does the structure of the alveoli make gas exchange efficient?

6. How is oxygen carried in the blood?

7. List the structures that air passes on its way from the nose to the alveoli:

8. What is the function of the mucus and cilia lining the respiratory passages?

9. How do movements of the ribs and diaphragm bring about inspiration? Circle the correct statement below.

    a) The diaphragm domes up into the thorax and ribs move in and down

b) The diaphragm flattens and ribs move up and out

c) The diaphragm domes up into the thorax and the ribs move up and out.

d) The diaphragm flattens and the ribs move in and down

10. What is the function of the epiglottis?

11. What controls the rate of breathing?

Test Yourself Answers

Websites

- http://www.biotopics.co.uk/humans/resyst.html Bio topics

A good interactive explanation of breathing and gas exchange in humans with diagrams to label, animations to watch and questions to answer.

- http://www.schoolscience.co.uk/content/4/biology/abpi/asthma/asth3.html School Science

Although this is of the human respiratory system there is a good diagram that gives the functions of the various parts as you move your mouse over it. Also an animation of gas exchange and a quiz to test your understanding of it.

- http://en.wikipedia.org/wiki/Lung Wikipedia

Wikipedia on the lungs. Lots of good information on the human respiratory system with all sorts of links if you are interested.

Glossary

- Link to Glossary [4]

References

[1] http://flickr.com/photos/daisy2/661821348/
[2] http://www.wikieducator.org/Respiratory_System_Worksheet

Anatomy and Physiology of Animals/Respiratory System/Test Yourself Answers

1. What is meant by the phrase "gas exchange"?

    Gas exchange is the addition of oxygen to the blood and the removal of carbon dioxide.

2. Where does gas exchange take place?

    Gas exchange takes place in the *alveoli of the lungs*.

3. What is the process by which oxygen moves from the alveoli into the blood?

    Oxygen moves from the alveoli into the blood by *diffusion*.

4. Why does this process occur?

    This process occurs because oxygen is at a much higher concentration in the alveoli than in the blood. Diffusion always occurs from a high to low concentration.

5. How does the structure of the alveoli make gas exchange efficient?

    The thin walls of the alveoli and the capillaries give only a small distance for the oxygen and carbon dioxide to diffuse across making gas exchange efficient.

    6. How is oxygen carried in the blood?

    Oxygen is carried in the blood combined with haemoglobin in the red blood cells.

7. List the structures that air passes on its way from the nose to the alveoli:

    On its way to the alveoli of the lungs air travels through the nasal cavity, pharynx, larynx, trachea, bronchi and bronchioles.

8. What is the function of the mucous and cilia lining the respiratory passages?

    The mucus and cilia in the respiratory passages trap dust particles and transport them to the mouth and nose for expulsion.

9. How do movements of the ribs and diaphragm bring about inspiration? Circle the correct statement below.

    b) *The diaphragm flattens and ribs move up and out.*

10. What is the function of the epiglottis?

    The epiglottis closes the larynx during swallowing so that food cannot enter the trachea.

11. What controls the rate of breathing?

    The concentration of carbon dioxide in the blood controls the rate of breathing.

Anatomy and Physiology of Animals/Lymphatic System

Objectives

After completing this section, you should know:

- the function of the lymphatic system
- what the terms tissue fluid, lymph, lymphocyte and lymphatic mean
- how lymph is formed and what is in it
- the basic structure and function of a lymph node and the position of some important lymph nodes in the body
- the route by which lymph circulates in the body and is returned to the blood system
- the location and function of the spleen, thymus and lacteals

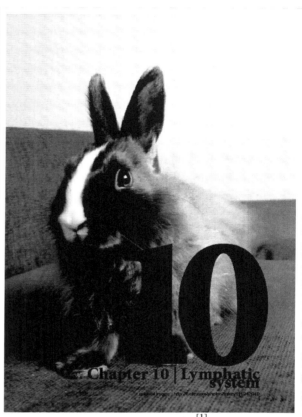

Lymphatic System

When **tissue fluid** enters the small blind-ended **lymphatic capillaries** that form a network between the cells it becomes **lymph**. Lymph is a clear watery fluid that is very similar to blood plasma except that it contains large numbers of white blood cells, mostly **lymphocytes**. It also contains protein, cellular debris, foreign particles and bacteria. Lymph that comes from the intestines also contains many fat globules following the absorption of fat from the digested food into the lymphatics (**lacteals**) of the villi (see chapter 11 for more on these). From the lymph capillaries the lymph flows into larger tubes called **lymphatic vessels.** These carry the lymph back to join the blood circulation (see diagrams 10.1 and 10.2).

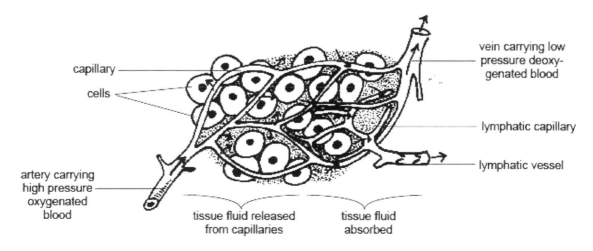

Diagram 10.1 - A capillary bed with lymphatic capillaries

Lymphatic vessels

Lymphatic vessels have several similarities to veins. Both are thin walled and return fluid to the right hand side of the heart. The movement of the fluid in both is brought about by the contraction of the muscles that surround them and both have valves to prevent backflow. One important difference is that lymph passes through at least one **lymph node** or gland before it reaches the blood system (see diagram 10.2). These filter out used cell parts, cancer cells and bacteria and help defend the body from infection.

Lymph nodes are of various sizes and shapes and found throughout the body and the more important ones are shown in diagram 10.3. They consist of lymph tissue surrounded by a fibrous sheath. Lymph flows into them through a number of incoming vessels. It then trickles through small channels where white cells called **macrophages** (derived from **monocytes**) remove the bacteria and debris by engulfing and digesting them (see diagram 10.4). The lymph then leaves the lymph nodes through outgoing vessels to continue its journey towards the heart where it rejoins the blood circulation (see diagrams 10.2 and 10.3).

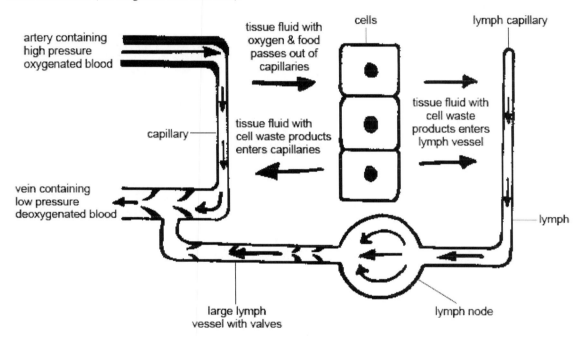

Diagram 10.2 - The lymphatic system

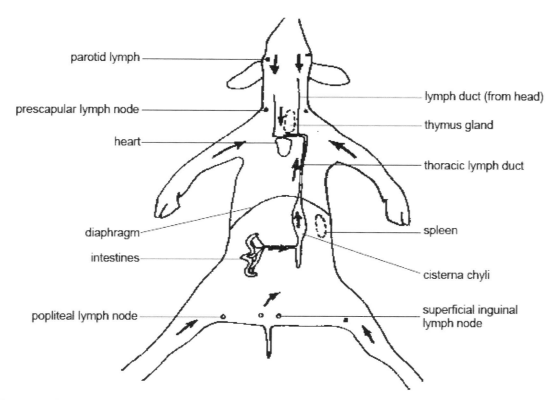

Diagram 10.3 - The circulation of lymph with major lymph nodes

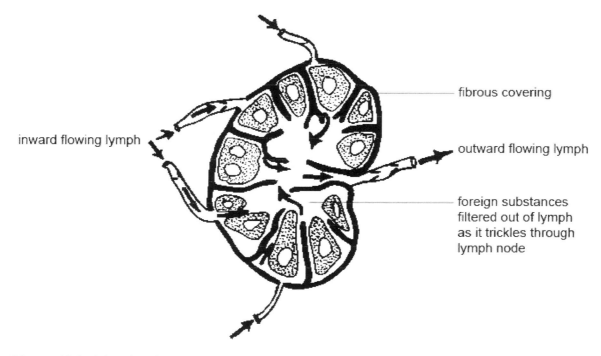

Diagram 10.4 - A lymph node

As well as filtering the lymph, lymph nodes produce the white cells known as **lymphocytes**. Lymphocytes are also produced by the **thymus**, **spleen** and **bone marrow**. There are two kinds of lymphocyte. The first attach invading micro organisms directly while others produce **antibodies** that circulate in the blood and attack them.

The function of the lymphatic system can therefore be summarized as transport and defense. It is important for returning the fluid and proteins that have escaped from the blood capillaries to the blood system and is also responsible for picking up the products of fat digestion in the small intestine. Its other essential function is as part of the immune system, defending the body against infection.

Problems with lymph nodes and the lymphatic system

During infection of the body the lymph nodes often become swollen and tender because of their increased activity. This is what causes the swollen 'glands' in your neck during throat infections, mumps and tonsillitis. Sometimes the bacteria multiply in the lymph node and cause inflammation. Cancer cells may also be carried to the lymph nodes and then transported to other parts of the body where they may multiply to form a secondary growth or **metastasis**. The lymphatic system may therefore contribute to the spread of cancer. Inactivity of the muscles surrounding the lymphatic vessels or blockage of these vessels causes tissue fluid to 'back up' in the tissues resulting in swelling or **oedema**.

Other Organs Of The Lymphatic System

The **spleen** is an important part of the lymphatic system. It is a deep red organ situated in the abdomen caudal to the stomach (see diagram 10.3). It is composed of two different types of tissue. The first type makes and stores lymphocytes, the cells of the immune system. The second type of tissue destroys worn out red blood cells, breaking down the haemoglobin into iron, which is recycled, and waste products that are excreted. The spleen also stores red blood cells. When severe blood loss occurs, it contracts and releases them into the circulation.

The **thymus** is a large pink organ lying just under the sternum (breastbone) just cranial to the heart (see diagram 10.1). It has an important function processing lymphocytes so they are capable of recognising and attacking foreign invaders like bacteria.

Other lymph organs are the **bone marrow** of the long bones where lymphocytes are produced and **lymph nodules**, which are like tiny lymph nodes. Large clusters of these are found in the wall of the small intestine (called Peyer's Patches) and in the tonsils.

Summary

- Fluid leaks out of the thin walled capillaries as they pass through the tissues. This is called **tissue fluid**.
- Much of tissue fluid passes back into the capillaries. Some enters the blind-ended lymphatic capillaries that form a network between the cells of the tissues. This fluid is called **lymph**.
- Lymph flows from the **lymphatic capillaries** to **lymph vessels**, passing through **lymph nodes** and along the thoracic duct to join the blood system.
- Lymph nodes filter the lymph and produce **lymphocytes**.
- Other organs of the lymphatic system are the **spleen, thymus, bone marrow**, and **lymph nodules**.

Worksheets

Lymphatic System Worksheet [2]

Test Yourself

1. What is the difference between tissue fluid and lymph?

2. By what route does lymph make its way back to join the blood of the circulatory system?

3. As the lymphatic system has no heart to push the lymph along what makes it flow?

4. What happens to the lymph as it passes through a lymph node?

5. Where is the spleen located in the body?

6. Where is the thymus located in the body?

7. What is the function of lymphocytes?

Test Yourself Answers

Websites

- http://www.cancerhelp.org.uk/help/default.asp?page=117 Cancerhelp

A nice clear explanation here with great diagrams of the (human) lymphatic system.

- http://www.jdaross.cwc.net/lymphatics2.htm Lymphatic system

Introduction to the Lymphatic System. A good description of lymph circulation with an animation.

- http://en.wikipedia.org/wiki/Lymphatic_system Wikipedia

Good information here on the (human) lymphatic system, lymph circulation and lymphoid organs.

Glossary

- Link to Glossary [4]

References

[1] http://flickr.com/photos/toms/111942949
[2] http://www.wikieducator.org/Lymphatic_System_Worksheet

Anatomy and Physiology of Animals/Lymphatic System/Test Yourself Answers

1. What is the difference between tissue fluid and lymph? *Tissue fluid is the fluid that has leaked out of the capillaries into the spaces around the cells of the tissues. Lymph is tissue fluid that has entered the lymphatic system i.e. the difference is largely one of location.*

2. By what route does lymph make its way back to join the blood of the circulatory system? *Lymph makes it way back to join the blood in the circulatory system via the lymphatic capillaries, lymphatic vessels, at least one lymph node and the thoracic duct. The lymph then joins the blood in veins that carry it back to the heart.*

3. As the lymphatic system has no heart to push the lymph along what makes it flow? *As the lymphatic system has no heart to push the lymph along it is pushed along mainly by the contraction of skeletal muscles that lie alongside the lymphatics.*

4. What happens to the lymph as it passes through a lymph node? *As the lymph passes through a lymph node, bacteria and debris are filtered from it and lymphocytes are added to it.*

5. Where is the spleen located in the body? *The spleen is found in the abdomen alongside and slightly caudal to the stomach.*

6. Where is the thymus located in the body? The thymus gland is located in the thorax beneath the sternum and just cranial to the heart.

7. What is the function of lymphocytes? *Lymphocytes defend the body from invasion by microorganisms. Some attach to the organisms directly while others produce antibodies that circulate in the blood and attack them.*

Anatomy and Physiology of Animals/The Gut and Digestion

Objectives

After completing this section, you should know:

- what is meant by the terms: ingestion, digestion, absorption, assimilation, egestion, peristalsis and chyme
- the characteristics, advantages and disadvantages of a herbivorous, carnivorous and omnivorous diet
- the 4 main functions of the gut
- the parts of the gut in the order in which the food passes down it

The Gut And Digestion

Plant cells are made of organic molecules using energy from the sun. This process is called **photosynthesis**. Animals rely on these ready-made organic molecules to supply them with their food. Some animals (herbivores) eat plants; some (carnivores) eat the herbivores.

Herbivores

Although **herbivores** eat plant material they have a basic problem. Their own digestive enzymes do not break down the large **cellulose** molecules in the plant cell walls. **Micro-organisms** like bacteria, on the other hand, can break them down. Therefore herbivores employ micro-organisms to do the job for them.

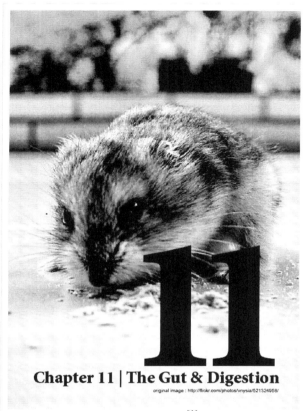

Chapter 11 | The Gut & Digestion

original image : http://flickr.com/photos/vnysia/521324958/

original image by vnysia [1] cc by

There are two types of herbivore:

> The first, **ruminants** like cattle, sheep and goats, house these bacteria in a special compartment in the enlarged stomach called the **rumen**.

> The second group has an enlarged large intestine and caecum, called a **functional caecum**, occupied

by cellulose digesting micro-organisms. These non-ruminant herbivores include the horse, rabbit and rat.

Even with the help of microorganisms, eating plants still poses problems. Plants are not a good source of nutrients, and herbivores have to eat large quantities of food to obtain all they require. Herbivores like cows, horses and rabbits typically spend much of their day feeding. To give the micro- organisms access to the cellulose molecules, the plant cell walls need to be broken down. This is why herbivores have teeth that are adapted to crush and grind. Their guts also tend to be lengthy and the food takes a long time to pass through it.

Eating plants does have some advantages. Plants are immobile so herbivores normally have to spend little energy collecting them. This contrasts with the other main group of animals- the carnivores that often have to chase their prey.

Carnivores

Carnivorous animals like those in the cat and dog families, bears, seals, crocodiles and birds of prey catch and eat other animals. They often have to use large amounts of energy finding, stalking, catching and killing their prey. However, they are rewarded by the fact that meat provides a very concentrated source of nutrients. Carnivores in the wild therefore tend to eat distinct meals often with long and irregular intervals between them. Time after feeding is spent digesting and absorbing the food.

The guts of carnivores are usually shorter and less complex than those of herbivores because meat is easier to digest than plant material. Carnivores usually have teeth that are specialised for dealing with flesh, gristle and bone. They have sleek bodies, strong, sharp claws and keen senses of smell, hearing and sight. They are also often cunning, alert and have an aggressive nature.

Omnivores

Many animals feed on both animal and vegetable material – they are **omnivorous.** Most primates including humans belong to this category as do pigs and rats. Their food is diverse, ranging from plant material to animals they have either killed themselves or scavenged from other carnivores. Omnivores lack the specialised teeth and guts of carnivores and herbivores but are often highly intelligent and adaptable reflecting their varied diet.

Treatment Of Food

Whether an animal eats plants or flesh, the **carbohydrates**, **fats** and **proteins** in the food it eats are generally giant molecules (see chapter 1). These need to be split up into smaller ones before they can pass into the blood and enter the cells to be used for energy or to make new cell constituents.

For example:

> **Carbohydrates** like cellulose, starch, and glycogen need to be split into **glucose** and other **monosaccharides**;
>
> **Proteins** need to be split into **amino acids**;
>
> **Fats** or **lipids** need to be split into **fatty acids** and **glycerol**.

The Gut

The **digestive tract, alimentary canal** or **gut** is a hollow tube stretching from the mouth to the anus. It is the organ system concerned with the treatment of foods.

At the mouth the large food molecules are taken into the gut - this is called **ingestion**. They must then be broken down into smaller ones by digestive enzymes - **digestion**, before they can be taken from the gut into the blood stream - **absorption**. The cells of the body can then use these small molecules - **assimilation**. The indigestible waste products are eliminated from the body by the act of **egestion** (see diagram 11.1).

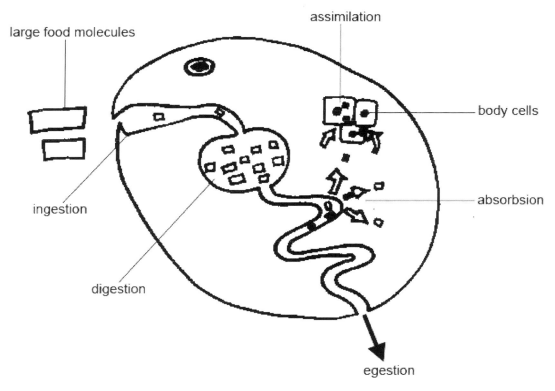

Diagram 11.1 - From ingestion to egestion

The 4 major functions of the gut are:

    1. Transporting the food;

    2. Processing the food physically by breaking it up (chewing), mixing, adding fluid etc.

    3. Processing the food chemically by adding digestive enzymes to split large food molecules into smaller ones.

    4. Absorbing these small molecules into the blood stream so the body can use them.

The regions of a typical mammals gut (for example a cat or dog) are shown in diagram 11.2.

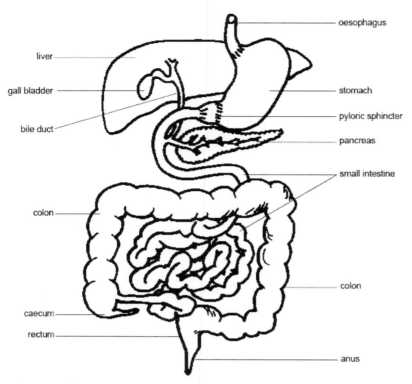

Diagram 11.2 - A typical mammalian gut

The food that enters the **mouth** passes to the **oesophagus**, then to the **stomach, small intestine, caecum, large intestine, rectum** and finally undigested material exits at the **anus**. The **liver** and **pancreas** produce secretions that aid digestion and the **gall bladder** stores **bile**.

Mouth

The mouth takes food into the body. The lips hold the food inside the mouth during chewing and allow the baby animal to suck on its mother's teat. In elephants the lips (and nose) have developed into the trunk which is the main food collecting tool. Some mammals, e.g. hamsters, have stretchy cheek pouches that they use to carry food or material to make their nests.

The sight or smell of food and its presence in the mouth stimulates the **salivary glands** to secrete **saliva**. There are four pairs of these glands in cats and dogs (see diagram 11.3). The fluid they produce moistens and softens the food making it easier to swallow. It also contains the enzyme, **salivary amylase**, which starts the digestion of starch.

The **tongue** moves food around the mouth and rolls it into a ball for swallowing. **Taste buds** are located on the tongue and in dogs and cats it is covered with spiny projections used for grooming and lapping. The cow's tongue is prehensile and wraps around grass to graze it.

Swallowing is a complex reflex involving 25 different muscles. It pushes food into the oesophagus and at the same time a small flap of tissue called the **epiglottis** closes off the windpipe so food doesn't go 'down the wrong way' and choke the animal (see diagram 11.4).

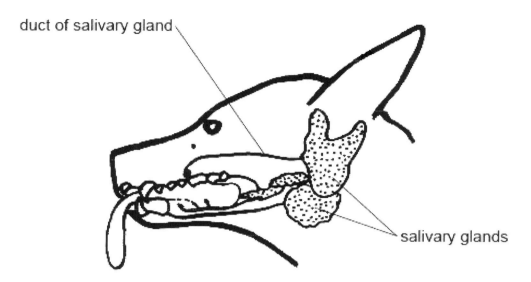

Diagram 11.3 - Salivary glands

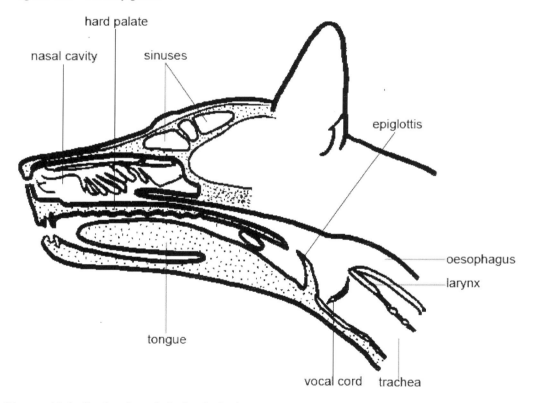

Diagram 11.4 - Section through the head of a dog

Teeth

Teeth seize, tear and grind food. They are inserted into sockets in the bone and consist of a crown above the gum and root below. The crown is covered with a layer of **enamel**, the hardest substance in the body. Below this is the **dentine**, a softer but tough and shock resistant material. At the centre of the tooth is a space filled with **pulp** which contains blood vessels and nerves. The tooth is cemented into the **socket** and in most teeth the tip of the root is quite narrow with a small opening for the blood vessels and nerves (see diagram 11.5).

In teeth that grow continuously, like the incisors of rodents, the opening remains large and these teeth are called **open rooted teeth**. Mammals have 2 distinct sets of teeth. The first the **milk teeth** are replaced by the **permanent teeth**.

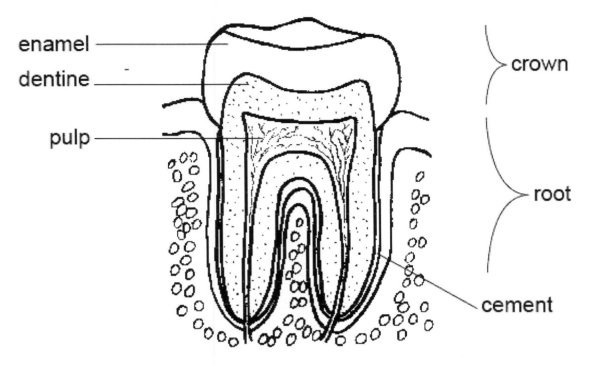

Diagram 11.5 - Structure of a tooth

Types Of Teeth

All the teeth of fish and reptiles are similar but mammals usually have four different types of teeth.

The **incisors** are the chisel-shaped 'biting off' teeth at the front of the mouth. In rodents and rabbits the incisors never stop growing (open-rooted teeth). They must be worn or ground down continuously by gnawing. They have hard enamel on one surface only so they wear unevenly and maintain their sharp cutting edge.

The largest incisors in the animal kingdom are found in elephants, for tusks are actually giant incisors. Sloths have no incisors at all, and sheep have no incisors in the upper jaw (see diagram 11.6). Instead there is a horny pad against which the bottom incisors cut.

The **canines** or 'wolf-teeth' are long, cone-shaped teeth situated just behind the incisors. They are particularly well developed in the dog and cat families where they are used to hold, stab and kill the prey (see diagram 11.7).

The tusks of boars and walruses are large canines while rodents and herbivores like sheep have no (or reduced) canines. In these animals the space where the canines would normally be is called the **diastema**. In rodents like the rat and beaver it allows the debris from gnawing to be expelled easily.

The cheek teeth or **premolars** and **molars** crush and grind the food. They are particularly well developed in herbivores where they have complex ridges that form broad grinding surfaces (see diagram 11.6). These are created from alternating bands of hard enamel and softer dentine that wear at different rates.

In carnivores the premolars and molars slice against each other like scissors and are called **carnassial** teeth see diagram 11.7). They are used for shearing flesh and bone.

Dental Formula

The numbers of the different kinds of teeth can be expressed in a **dental formula**. This gives the numbers of incisors, canines, premolars and molars in **one half** of the mouth. The numbers of these four types of teeth in the left **or** right **half of the upper jaw** are written above a horizontal line and the four types of teeth in the right **or** left **half of the lower jaw** are written below it.

Thus the dental formula for the sheep is:

0.0.3.3

3.1.3.3

It indicates that in the upper right (or left) **half** of the jaw there are no incisors or canines (i.e. there is a **diastema**), three premolars and three molars. In the lower right (or left) **half** of the jaw are three incisors, one canine, three premolars and three molars (see diagram 11.6).

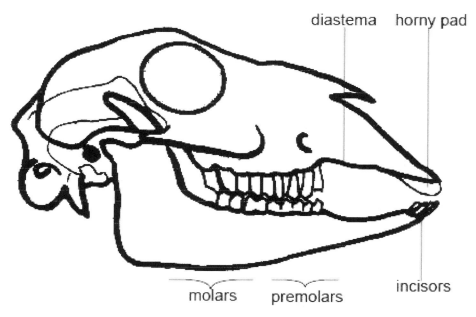

diastema   horny pad

molars   premolars   incisors

Diagram 11.6 - A sheep's skull

The dental formula for a dog is:

3.1.4.2

3.1.4.3

The formula indicates that in the right (or left) **half** of the upper jaw there are three incisors, one canine, four premolars and two molars. In the right (or left) **half** of the lower jaw there are three incisors, one canine, four premolars and three molars (see diagram 11.7).

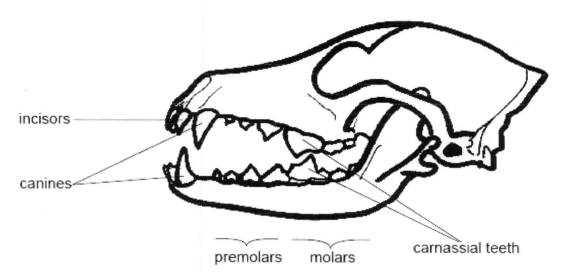

incisors

canines

premolars   molars

carnassial teeth

Diagram 11.7 - A dog's skull

Oesophagus

The **oesophagus** transports food to the stomach. Food is moved along the oesophagus, as it is along the small and large intestines, by contraction of the smooth muscles in the walls that push the food along rather like toothpaste along a tube. This movement is called **peristalsis** (see diagram 11.8).

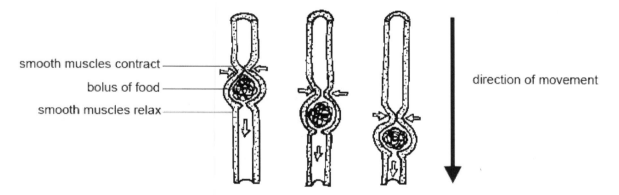

smooth muscles contract

bolus of food

smooth muscles relax

direction of movement

Diagram 11.8 - Peristalsis

Stomach

The **stomach** stores and mixes the food. Glands in the wall secrete **gastric juice** that contains enzymes to digest protein and fats as well as **hydrochloric acid** to make the contents very acidic. The walls of the stomach are very muscular and churn and mix the food with the gastric juice to form a watery mixture called **chyme** (pronounced kime). Rings of muscle called **sphincters** at the entrance and exit to the stomach control the movement of food into and out of it (see diagram 11.9).

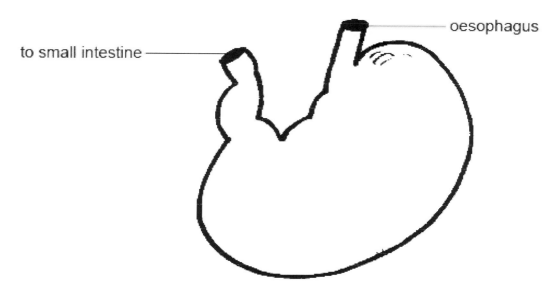

Diagram 11.9 - The stomach

Small Intestine

Most of the breakdown of the large food molecules and absorption of the smaller molecules take place in the long and narrow small intestine. The total length varies but it is about 6.5 metres in humans, 21 metres in the horse, 40 metres in the ox and over 150 metres in the blue whale.

It is divided into 3 sections: the duodenum (after the stomach), jejunum and ileum. The duodenum receives 3 different secretions:

1) **Bile** from the liver;

2) **Pancreatic juice** from the pancreas and

3) **Intestinal juice** from glands in the intestinal wall.

These complete the digestion of starch, fats and protein. The products of digestion are absorbed into the blood and lymphatic system through the wall of the intestine, which is lined with tiny finger-like projections called **villi** that increase the surface area for more efficient absorption (see diagram 11.10).

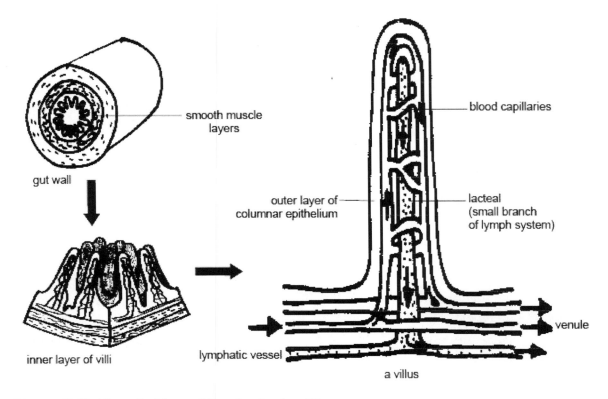

Diagram 11.10 - The wall of the small intestine showing villi

The Rumen

In ruminant herbivores like cows, sheep and antelopes the stomach is highly modified to act as a "fermentation vat". It is divided into four parts. The largest part is called the **rumen**. In the cow it occupies the entire left half of the abdominal cavity and can hold up to 270 litres. The **reticulum** is much smaller and has a honeycomb of raised folds on its inner surface. In the camel the reticulum is further modified to store water. The next part is called the **omasum** with a folded inner surface. Camels have no omasum. The final compartment is called the **abomasum**. This is the 'true' stomach where muscular walls churn the food and gastric juice is secreted (see diagram 11.11).

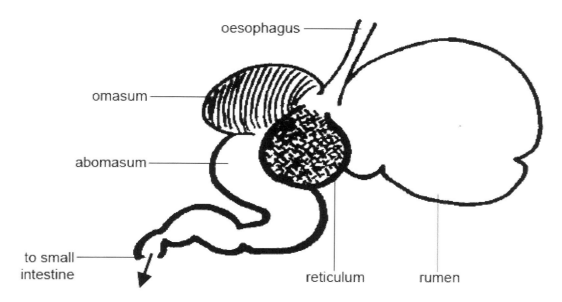

Diagram 11.11 - The rumen

Ruminants swallow the grass they graze almost without chewing and it passes down the oesophagus to the rumen and reticulum. Here liquid is added and the muscular walls churn the food. These chambers provide the main fermentation vat of the ruminant stomach. Here bacteria and single-celled animals start to act on the cellulose plant cell walls. These organisms break down the cellulose to smaller molecules that are absorbed to provide the cow or sheep with energy. In the process, the gases methane and carbon dioxide are produced. These cause the "burps" you may hear cows and sheep making.

Not only do the micro-organisms break down the cellulose but they also produce the **vitamins E, B and K** for use by the animal. Their digested bodies provide the ruminant with the majority of its protein requirements.

In the wild grazing is a dangerous activity as it exposes the herbivore to predators. They crop the grass as quickly as possible and then when the animal is in a safer place the food in the rumen can be regurgitated to be chewed at the animal's leisure. This is 'chewing the cud' or **rumination**. The finely ground food may be returned to the rumen for further work by the microorganisms or, if the particles are small enough, it will pass down a special groove in the wall of the oesophagus straight into the omasum. Here the contents are kneaded and water is absorbed before they pass to the abomasum. The abomasum acts as a "proper" stomach and gastric juice is secreted to digest the protein.

Large Intestine

The **large intestine** consists of the **caecum, colon** and **rectum**. The chyme from the small intestine that enters the colon consists mainly of water and undigested material such as cellulose (fibre or roughage). In omnivores like the pig and humans the main function of the colon is absorption of water to give solid faeces. Bacteria in this part of the gut produce vitamins B and K.

The caecum, which forms a dead-end pouch where the small intestine joins the large intestine, is small in pigs and humans and helps water absorption. However, in rabbits, rodents and horses, the caecum is very large and called the **functional caecum**. It is here that cellulose is digested by micro-organisms. The **appendix**, a narrow dead end tube at the end of the caecum, is particularly large in primates but seems to have no digestive function.

Functional Caecum

The caecum in the rabbit, rat and guinea pig is greatly enlarged to provide a "fermentation vat" for micro-organisms to break down the cellulose plant cell walls. This is called a **functional caecum** (see diagram 11.12). In the horse both the caecum and the colon are enlarged. As in the rumen, the large cellulose molecules are broken down to smaller molecules that can be absorbed. However, the position of the functional caecum after the main areas of digestion and absorption, means it is potentially less effective than the rumen. This means that the small molecules that are produced there can not be absorbed by the gut but pass out in the faeces. The rabbit and rodents (and foals) solve this problem by eating their own faeces so that they pass through the gut a second time and the products of cellulose digestion can be absorbed in the small intestine. Rabbits produce two kinds of faeces. Softer night-time faeces are eaten directly from the anus and the harder pellets you are probably familiar with, that have passed through the gut twice.

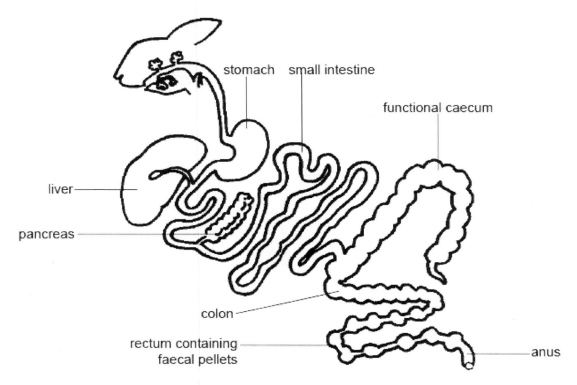

Diagram 11.12 - The gut of a rabbit

The Gut Of Birds

Birds' guts have important differences from mammals' guts. Most obviously, birds have a **beak** instead of teeth. Beaks are much lighter than teeth and are an adaptation for flight. Imagine a bird trying to take off and fly with a whole set of teeth in its head! At the base of the oesophagus birds have a bag-like structure called a **crop**. In many birds the crop stores food before it enters the stomach, while in pigeons and doves glands in the crop secretes a special fluid called **crop-milk** which parent birds regurgitate to feed their young. The stomach is also modified and consists of two compartments. The first is the true stomach with muscular walls and enzyme secreting glands. The second compartment is the **gizzard**. In seed eating birds this has very muscular walls and contains pebbles swallowed by the bird to help grind the food. This is the reason why you must always supply a caged bird with grit. In birds of prey like the falcon the walls of the gizzard are much thinner and expand to accommodate large meals (see diagram 11.13).

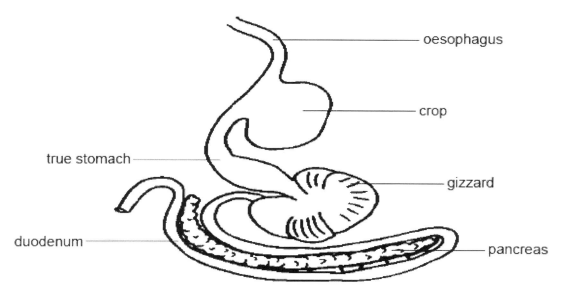

Diagram 11.13 - The stomach and small intestine of a hen

Digestion

During digestion the large food molecules are broken down into smaller molecules by **enzymes**. The three most important groups of enzymes secreted into the gut are:

1. **Amylases** that split carbohydrates like starch and glycogen into monosaccharides like glucose.
2. **Proteases** that split proteins into amino acids.
3. **Lipases** that split lipids or fats into fatty acids and glycerol.

Glands produce various secretions which mix with the food as it passes along the gut.

These secretions include:

1. **Saliva** secreted into the mouth from several pairs of **salivary glands** (see diagram 11.3). Saliva consists mainly of water but contains salts, mucous and salivary amylase. The function of saliva is to lubricate food as it is chewed and swallowed and salivary amylase begins the digestion of starch.
2. **Gastric juice** secreted into the stomach from glands in its walls. Gastric juice contains **pepsin** that breaks down protein and hydrochloric acid to produce the acidic conditions under which this enzyme works best. In baby animals rennin to digest milk is also produced in the stomach.
3. **Bile** produced by the liver. It is stored in the **gall bladder** and secreted into the duodenum via the **bile duct** (see diagram 11.14). (Note that the horse, deer, parrot and rat have no gall bladder). Bile is not a digestive enzyme. Its function is to break up large globules of fat into smaller ones so the fat splitting enzymes can gain access the fat molecules.

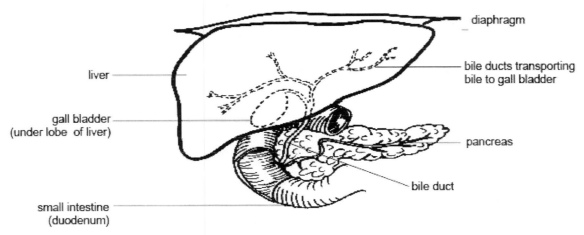

Diagram 11.14 - The liver, gall bladder and pancreas

Pancreatic juice

The **pancreas** is a gland located near the beginning of the duodenum (see diagram 11.14). In most animals it is large and easily seen but in rodents and rabbits it lies within the membrane linking the loops of the intestine (the **mesentery**) and is quite difficult to find. **Pancreatic juice** is produced in the pancreas. It flows into the duodenum and contains **amylase** for digesting starch, **lipase** for digesting fats and **protease** for digesting proteins.

Intestinal juice

Intestinal juice is produced by glands in the lining of the small intestine. It contains enzymes for digesting disaccharides and proteins as well as mucus and salts to make the contents of the small intestine more alkaline so the enzymes can work.

Absorption

The small molecules produced by digestion are absorbed into the **villi** of the wall of the **small intestine**. The tiny finger-like projections of the villi increase the surface area for absorption. Glucose and amino acids pass directly through the wall into the blood stream by diffusion or active transport. Fatty acids and glycerol enter vessels of the lymphatic system (**lacteals**) that run up the centre of each villus.

The Liver

The liver is situated in the abdominal cavity adjacent to the diaphragm (see diagrams 2 and 14). It is the largest single organ of the body and has over 100 known functions. Its most important digestive functions are:

1. the production of **bile** to help the digestion of fats (described above) and
2. the control of **blood sugar** levels

Glucose is absorbed into the capillaries of the villi of the intestine. The blood stream takes it directly to the liver via a blood vessel known as the **hepatic portal vessel** or **vein** (see diagram 11.15).

The liver converts this glucose into glycogen which it stores. When glucose levels are low the liver can convert the glycogen back into glucose. It releases this back into the blood to keep the level of glucose constant. The hormone **insulin**, produced by special cells in the **pancreas**, controls this process.

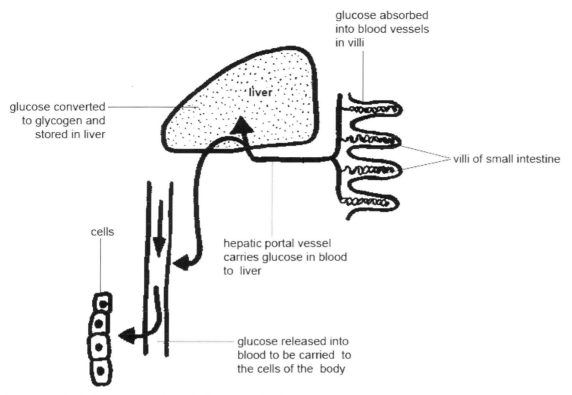

glucose absorbed
into blood vessels
in villi

glucose converted
to glycogen and
stored in liver

villi of small intestine

cells

hepatic portal vessel
carries glucose in blood
to liver

glucose released into
blood to be carried to
the cells of the body

Diagram 11.15 - The control of blood glucose by the liver

Other functions of the liver include:

3. making **vitamin A**,

4. making the **proteins** that are found in the **blood plasma (albumin, globulin** and **fibrinogen)**,

5. storing **iron**,

6. removing **toxic substances** like alcohol and poisons from the blood and converting them to safer substances,

7. producing **heat** to help maintain the temperature of the body.

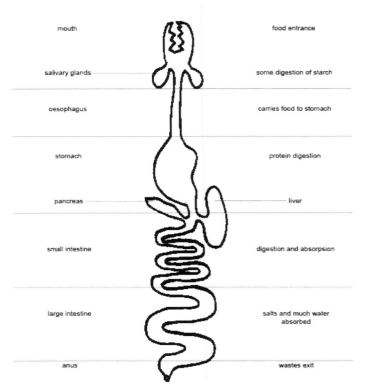

mouth	food entrance
salivary glands	some digestion of starch
oesophagus	carries food to stomach
stomach	protein digestion
pancreas	liver
small intestine	digestion and absorpsion
large intestine	salts and much water absorbed
anus	wastes exit

Diagram 11.16 - Summary of the main functions of the different regions of the gut

Summary

- The **gut** breaks down plant and animal materials into nutrients that can be used by animals' bodies.
- Plant material is more difficult to break down than animal tissue. The gut of **herbivores** is therefore longer and more complex than that of **carnivores**. Herbivores usually have a compartment (the **rumen** or **functional caecum**) housing micro-organisms to break down the **cellulose** wall of plants.
- Chewing by the teeth begins the food processing. There are 4 main types of teeth: **incisors, canines, premolars** and **molars**. In dogs and cats the premolars and molars are adapted to slice against each other and are called **carnassial** teeth.
- **Saliva** is secreted in the mouth. It lubricates the food for swallowing and contains an enzyme to break down starch.
- Chewed food is swallowed and passes down the **oesophagus** by waves of contraction of the wall called **peristalsis.** The food passes to the stomach where it is churned and mixed with acidic **gastric juice** that begins the digestion of protein.
- The resulting **chyme** passes down the small intestine where enzymes that digest fats, proteins and carbohydrates are secreted. **Bile** produced by the liver is also secreted here. It helps in the breakdown of fats. **Villi** provide the large surface area necessary for the absorption of the products of digestion.
- In the **colon** and **caecum** water is absorbed and micro organisms produce some **vitamin B and K**. In rabbits, horses and rodents the caecum is enlarged as a **functional caecum** and micro-organisms break down cellulose cell walls to simpler carbohydrates. Waste products exit the body via the **rectum** and **anus**.
- The **pancreas** produces **pancreatic juice** that contains many of the enzymes secreted into the small intestine.
- In addition to producing bile the liver regulates blood sugar levels by converting glucose absorbed by the villi into glycogen and storing it. The liver also removes toxic substances from the blood, stores iron, makes vitamin A and produces heat.

Worksheet

Use the Digestive System Worksheet [2] to help you learn the different parts of the digestive system and their functions.

Test Yourself

Then work through the Test Yourself below to see if you have understood and remembered what you learned.

1. Name the four different kinds of teeth

2. Give 2 facts about how the teeth of cats and dogs are adapted for a carnivorous diet:

    1.

    2.

3. What does saliva do to the food?

4. What is peristalsis?

5. What happens to the food in the stomach?

6. What is chyme?

7. Where does the chyme go after leaving the stomach?

8. What are villi and what do they do?

9. What happens in the small intestine?

10. Where is the pancreas and what does it do?

11. How does the caecum of rabbits differ from that of cats?

12. How does the liver help control the glucose levels in the blood?

13. Give 2 other functions of the liver:

    1.

    2.

Test Yourself Answers

Websites

- http://www.second-opinions.co.uk/carn_herb_comparison.html Second opinion. A good comparison of the guts of carnivores and herbivores

- http://www.chu.cam.ac.uk/~ALRF/giintro.htm The gastrointestinal system. A good comparison of the guts of carnivores and herbivores with more advanced information than in the previous site.

- http://www.westga.edu/~lkral/peristalsis/index.html Peristalsis animation.

- http://en.wikipedia.org/wiki/Digestion Wikipedia on digestion with links to further information on most aspects. Like most websites this is mainly about human digestion but much is applicable to animals.

Glossary

- Link to Glossary [4]

References

[1] http://flickr.com/photos/vnysia/521324958/
[2] http://www.wikieducator.org/Digestive_System_Worksheet

Anatomy and Physiology of Animals/The Gut and Digestion/Test Yourself Answers

1. Name the four different kinds of teeth

   The four different kinds of teeth are incisors, canines, premolars and molars.

2. Give 2 facts about how the teeth of cats and dogs are adapted for a carnivorous diet

   The teeth of cats and dogs are adapted for a carnivorous diet with small chisel shaped incisors for biting off flesh, sharp canines for holding and killing prey and carnassials for shearing flesh.

3. What does saliva do to the food?

   Saliva lubricates food for swallowing and contains an enzyme for breaking down starch.

4. What is peristalsis?

   Peristalsis is the waves of smooth muscle contraction that pass down the gut and move the food along.

5. What happens to the food in the stomach?

   In the stomach food is churned and mixed and gastric juice that contains enzymes to digest proteins is added. Hydrochloric acid to make the stomach contents acidic for the protein digesting enzymes is also added here.

6. What is chyme?

   Chyme is the liquefied and partially digested food that passes down the gut.

7. Where does the chyme go after leaving the stomach?

   The chyme enters the small intestine after leaving the stomach.

8. What are villi and what do they do?

   Villi are the small finger-like projections from the wall of the small intestine that increase the surface area for the absorption into the blood of the digested nutrients.

9. What happens in the small intestine?

   In the small intestine food is digested and resulting nutrients are absorbed into the blood via the villi.

10. Where is the pancreas and what does it do?

    The pancreas is situated in the first bend of the duodenum after it leaves the stomach. It produces pancreatic juice that contains enzymes for digesting carbohydrates, fats and proteins.

11. How does the caecum of rabbits differ from that of cats?

    In rabbits the caecum is enlarged to form a functional caecum that contains microorganisms for breaking down the cellulose walls of plants. Note that because of the position of the functional caecum at the end of the gut animals like the rabbit eat their faeces to take advantage of the digested nutrients.

12. How does the liver help control the glucose levels in the blood?

The liver helps control the glucose levels in the blood by converting the glucose to glycogen that it stores. This is then released when blood glucose levels are low. The hormone insulin produced by the pancreas controls this process.

13. Give 2 other functions of the liver

Other functions of the liver include the detoxification of toxic substances like alcohol, storing iron and production of bile, proteins, vitamin A and heat.

Anatomy and Physiology of Animals/Urinary System

Objectives

After completing this section, you should know:

- the parts of the urinary system
- the structure and function of a kidney
- the structure and function of a kidney tubule or nephron
- the processes of filtration, reabsorption, secretion and concentration that convert blood to urine in the kidney tubule
- the function of antidiuretic hormone in producing concentrated urine
- the composition, storage and voiding of normal urine
- abnormal constituents of urine and their significance
- the functions of the kidney in excreting nitrogenous waste, controlling water levels and regulating salt concentrations and acid-base balance
- that birds do not have a bladder

Chapter 12 | Urinary system

original image : http://flickr.com/photos/fazen/2615416/

original image by fazen [1] cc by

Homeostasis

The cells of an animal can only remain healthy if the conditions are just right. The processes that take place in them are upset if the temperature is too high or too low, or if the fluid around or inside them is too acid or alkaline. **Homeostasis** is the name given to the processes that help keep the internal conditions constant even when external conditions change. The word means, "staying the same".

There are a number of organs in the body that play a part in maintaining homeostasis. For example, the skin helps keep the internal temperature of bird and mammals bodies within a narrow range even when the outside temperatures change (see Chapters 5 and 16); the lungs control the amount of carbon dioxide in the blood (see Chapters 8 and 16); the liver and pancreas work together to keep the amount of glucose in the blood within narrow limits (see Chapter 5) and the kidneys regulate the acidity and the concentration of water and salt in the blood (also see Chapter 16). How the kidneys do this will be described later in this chapter.

Hormones are chemicals that carry messages around the body in the blood and are central to many of the homeostatic processes mentioned above. Their role will be described in more detail in Chapter 16.

Water In The Body

Water is essential for living things to survive because all the chemical reactions within a body take place in a solution of water. An animal's body consists of up to 80% water. The exact proportion depends on the type of animal, its age, sex, health and whether or not it has had sufficient to drink. Generally animals do not survive a loss of more than 15% of their body water.

In vertebrates almost 2/3rd of this water is in the cells (**intracellular fluid**). The rest is outside the cells (**extracellular fluid**) where it is found in the spaces around the cells (**tissue fluid**), as well as in the blood and lymph.

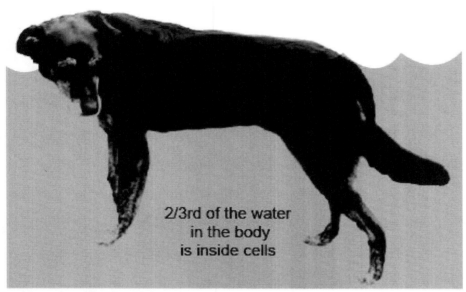

Diagram 12.1 - Water in the body

Maintaining Water Balance

Animals lose water through their skin and lungs, in the faeces and urine. These losses must be made up by water in food and drink and from the water that is a by-product of chemical reactions. If the animal does not manage to compensate for water loss the dissolved substances in the blood may become so concentrated they become lethal. To prevent this happening various mechanisms come into play as soon as the concentration of the blood increases. A part of the brain called the **hypothalamus** is in charge of these homeostatic processes. The most important is the feeling of thirst that is triggered by an increase in blood concentration. This stimulates an animal to find water and drink it.

The kidneys are also involved in maintaining water balance as various hormones instruct them to produce more concentrated urine and so retain some of the water that would otherwise be lost (see later in this Chapter and Chapter 16).

Desert Animals

Coping with water loss is a particular problem for animals that live in dry conditions. Some, like the camel, have developed great tolerance for dehydration. For example, under some conditions, camels can withstand the loss of one third of their body mass as water. They can also survive wide daily changes in temperature. This means they do not have to use large quantities of water in sweat to cool the body by evaporation.

Smaller animals are more able than large ones to avoid extremes of temperature or dry conditions by resting in sheltered more humid situations during the day and being active only at night.

The kangaroo rat is able to survive without access to any drinking water at all because it does not sweat and produces extremely concentrated urine. Water from its food and from chemical processes is sufficient to supply all its requirements.

Excretion

Animals need to excrete because they take in substances that are excess to the body's requirements and many of the chemical reactions in the body produce waste products. If these substances were not removed they would poison cells or slow down metabolism. All animals therefore have some means of getting rid of these wastes.

The major waste products in mammals are carbon dioxide that is removed by the lungs, and urea that is produced when excess amino acids (from proteins) are broken down. Urea is filtered from the blood by the kidneys.

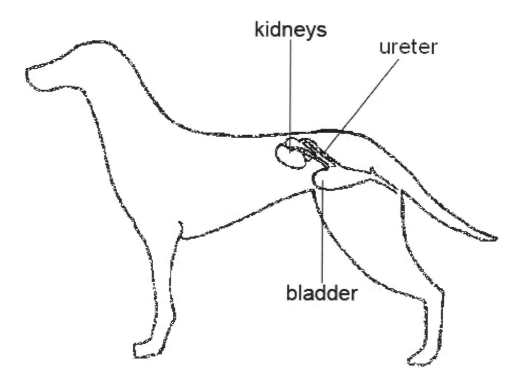

Diagram 12.2 - The position of the organs of the urinary system in a dog

The Kidneys And Urinary System

The **kidneys** in mammals are bean-shaped organs that lie in the abdominal cavity attached to the dorsal wall on either side of the spine (see diagram 12.2). An artery from the dorsal aorta called the **renal artery** supplies blood to them and the **renal vein** drains them.

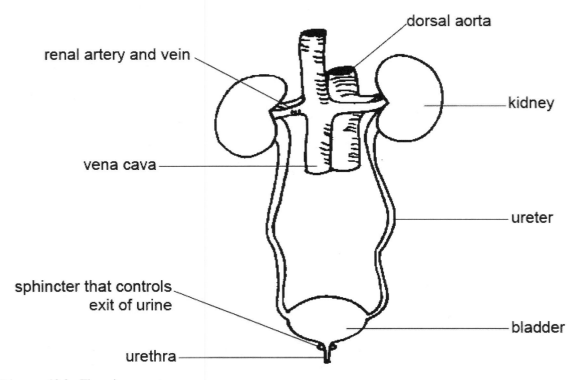

Diagram 12.3 - The urinary system

To the naked eye kidneys seem simple enough organs. They are covered by a fibrous coat or capsule and if cut in half lengthways (longitudinally) two distinct regions can be seen - an inner region or **medulla** and the outer **cortex**. A cavity within the kidney called the **pelvis** collects the urine and carries it to the **ureter**, which connects with the **bladder** where the urine is stored temporarily. Rings of muscle (**sphincters**) control the release of urine from the bladder and the urine leaves the body through the **urethra** (see diagrams 12.3 and 12.4).

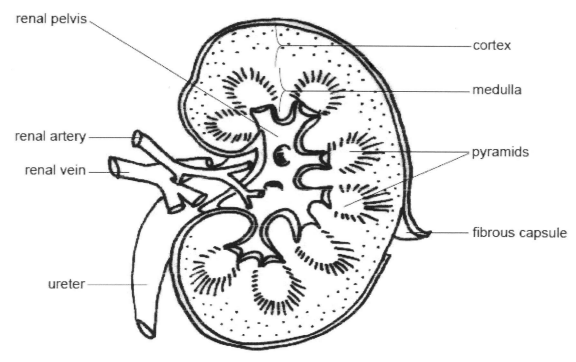

Diagram 12.4 - The dissected kidney

Kidney Tubules Or Nephrons

It is only when you examine kidneys under the microscope that you find that their structure is not simple at all. The cortex and medulla are seen to be composed of masses of tiny tubes. These are called **kidney tubules** or **nephrons** (see diagrams 12.5 and 12.6). A human kidney consists of over a million of them.

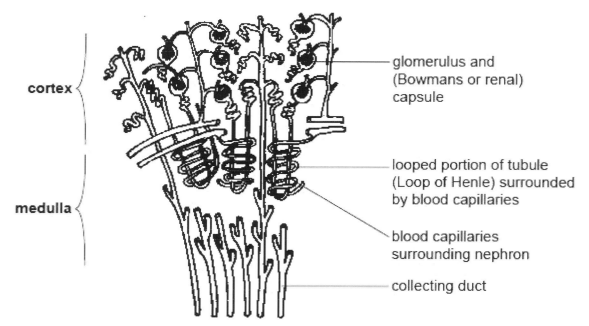

Diagram 12.5 - Several kidney tubules or nephrons

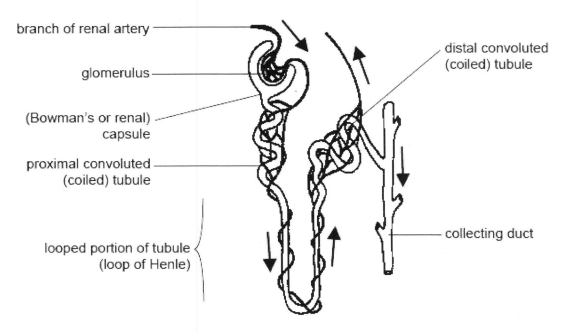

Diagram 12.6 - A kidney tubule or nephron

At one end of each nephron, in the cortex of the kidney, is a cup shaped structure called the (**Bowman's** or **renal**) **capsule**. It surrounds a tuft of capillaries called the **glomerulus** that carries high-pressure blood. Together the glomerulus and capsule act as a blood-filtering device (see diagram 12.7). The holes in the filter allow most of the contents of the blood through except the red and white cells and large protein molecules. The fluid flowing from the capsule into the rest of the kidney tubule is therefore very similar to blood plasma and contains many useful substances like water, glucose, salt and amino acids. It also contains waste products like **urea**.

Processes Occurring In The Nephron

After entering the glomerulus the filtered fluid flows along a coiled part of the tubule (the **proximal convoluted tubule**) to a looped portion (the **Loop of Henle**) and then to the **collecting tube** via a second length of coiled tube (the **distal convoluted tubule**) (see diagram 12.6). From the collecting ducts the urine flows into the **renal pelvis** and enters the **ureter**.

Note that the glomerulus, capsule and both coiled parts of the tubule are all situated in the cortex of the kidney while the loops of Henle and collecting ducts make up the medulla (see diagram 12.5).

As the fluid flows along the proximal convoluted tubule useful substances like glucose, water, salts, potassium ions, calcium ions and amino acids are **reabsorbed** into the blood capillaries that form a network around the tubules. Many of these substances are transported by active transport and energy is required.

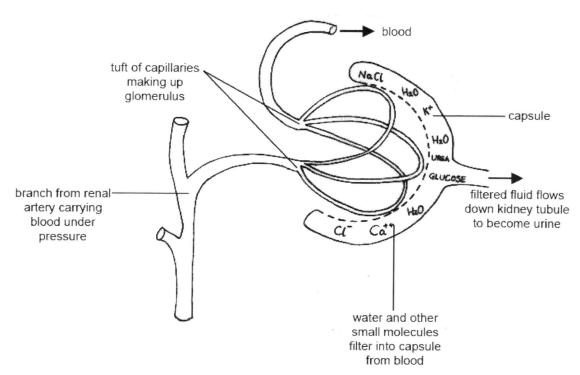

Diagram 12.7 - Filtration in the glomerulus and capsule

In a separate process, some substances, particularly potassium, ammonium and hydrogen ions, and drugs like penicillin, are actively **secreted** into the distal convoluted tubule.

By the time the fluid has reached the collecting ducts these processes of absorption and secretion have changed the fluid originally filtered into the Bowman's capsule into urine. The main function of the collecting ducts is then to remove more water from the urine if necessary. These processes are summarised in diagram 12.8.

Normal urine consists of water, in which waste products such as urea and salts such as sodium chloride are dissolved. Pigments from the breakdown of red blood cells give urine its yellow colour.

The Production Of Concentrated Urine

Because of the high pressure of the blood in the glomerulus and the large size of the pores in the glomerulus/capsule-filtering device, an enormous volume of fluid passes into the kidney tubules. If this fluid were left as it is, the animal's body would be drained dry in 30 minutes. In fact, as the fluid flows down the tubule, over 90% of the water in it is reabsorbed. The main part of this reabsorption takes place in the collecting tubes.

The amount of water removed from the collecting ducts is controlled by a hormone called **antidiuretic hormone (ADH)** produced by the **pituitary gland**, situated at the base of the brain. When the blood becomes more concentrated, as happens when an animal is deprived of water, ADH is secreted and causes more water to be absorbed from the collecting ducts so that concentrated urine is produced. When the animal has drunk plenty of water and the blood is dilute, no ADH is secreted and no or little water is absorbed from the collecting ducts, so dilute urine is produced. In this way the concentration of the blood is controlled precisely.

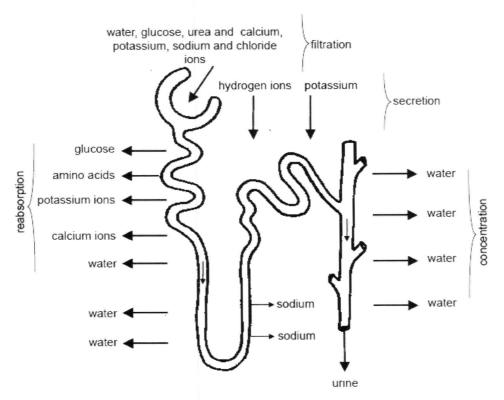

Diagram 12.8 - Summary of the processes involved in the formation of urine

Water Balance In Fish And Marine Animals

Fresh Water Fish

Although the skin of fish is more or less waterproof, the gills are very porous. The body fluids of fish that live in fresh water have a higher concentration of dissolved substances than the water in which they swim. In other words the body fluids of fresh water fish are **hypertonic** to the water (see chapter 3). Water therefore flows into the body by **osmosis**. To stop the body fluids being constantly diluted fresh water fish produce large quantities of dilute urine.

Marine Fish

Marine fish like the sharks and dogfish have body fluids that have the same concentration of dissolved substances as the water (**isotonic**) have little problem with water balance. However, marine bony fish like red cod, snapper and sole, have body fluids with a lower concentration of dissolved substances than seawater (they are **hypotonic** to seawater). This means that water tends to flow out of their bodies by osmosis. To make up this fluid loss they drink seawater and get rid of the excess salt by excreting it from the gills.

Marine Birds

Marine birds that eat marine fish take in large quantities of salt and some only have access to seawater for drinking. Bird's kidneys are unable to produce very concentrated urine, so they have developed a salt gland. This excretes a concentrated salt solution into the nose to get rid of the excess salt.

Diabetes And The Kidney

There are two types of diabetes. The most common is called sugar diabetes or **diabetes mellitus** and is common in cats and dogs especially if they are overweight. It is caused by the pancreas secreting insufficient **insulin**, the hormone that controls the amount of glucose in the blood. If insulin secretion is inadequate, the concentration of glucose in the blood increases. Any increase in the glucose in the blood automatically leads to an increase in glucose in the fluid filtered into the kidney tubule. Normally the kidney removes all the glucose filtered into it, but these high concentrations swamp this removal mechanism and urine containing glucose is produced. The main symptoms of this type of diabetes are the production of large amounts of dilute urine containing glucose, and excessive thirst.

The second type of diabetes is called **diabetes insipidus**. The name comes from the main symptom, which is the production of large amounts of very dilute and "tasteless" urine. It occurs when the pituitary gland produces insufficient ADH, the hormone that stimulates water re-absorption from the kidney tubule. When this hormone is lacking, water is not absorbed and large amounts of dilute urine are produced. Because so much water is lost in the urine, animals with this form of diabetes can die if deprived of water for only a day or so.

Other Functions Of The Kidney

The excretion of urea from the body and the maintenance of water balance, as described above, are the main functions of the kidney. However, the kidneys have other roles in keeping conditions in the body stable i.e. in maintaining homeostasis. These include:

- controlling the concentration of salt ions (Na+, K+, Cl-) in the blood by adjusting how much is excreted or retained;
- maintaining the correct acidity of the blood. Excess acid is constantly being produced by the normal chemical reactions in the body and the kidney eliminates this.

Normal Urine

Normal urine consists of water (95%), urea, salts (mostly sodium chloride) and pigments (mostly from bile) that give it its characteristic colour.

Abnormal Ingredients Of Urine

If the body is not working properly, small amounts of substances not normally present may be found in the urine or substances normally present may appear in abnormal amounts.

- The presence of **glucose** may indicate diabetes (see above).
- Urine with red blood cells in it is called **haematuria**, and may indicate inflammation of the kidney,or urinary tract, cancer or a blow to the kidneys.
- Sometimes free **haemoglobin** is found in the urine. This indicates that the red blood cells in the blood have **haemolysed** (the membrane has broken down) and the haemoglobin has passed into the kidney tubules.
- The presence of **white blood cells** in the urine indicates there is an infection in the kidney or urinary tract.
- **Protein molecules** are usually too large to pass into the kidney tubule so no or only small amounts of proteins like **albumin** is normally found in urine. Large quantities of albumin indicate that the kidney tubules have been injured or the kidney has become diseased. High blood pressure also pushes proteins from the blood into

the tubules.

- **Casts** are tiny cylinders of material that have been shed from the lining of the tubules and flushed out into the urine.
- **Mucus** is not usually found in the urine of healthy animals but is a normal constituent of horses' urine, giving it a characteristic cloudy appearance.

Tests can be carried out to identify any abnormal ingredients of urine. These tests are normally done by "**stix**", which are small plastic strips with absorbent ends impregnated with various chemicals. A colour change occurs in the presence of an abnormal ingredient.

Excretion In Birds

Birds' high body temperature and level of activity means that they need to conserve water. Birds therefore do not have a bladder and instead of excreting urea, which needs to be dissolved in large amounts of water, birds produce uric acid that can be discharged as a thick paste along with the feces. This is the white chalky part of the bird droppings that land on you or your car.

Summary

- The excretory system consists of paired **kidneys** and associated blood supply. **Ureters** transport urine from the kidneys to the bladder and the **urethra** with associated sphincter muscles controls the release of urine.
- The kidneys have an important role in maintaining **homeostasis** in the body. They excrete the waste product urea, control the concentrations of water and salt in the body fluids, and regulate the acidity of the blood.
- A kidney consists of an outer region or **cortex,** inner **medulla** and a cavity called the **pelvis** that collects the urine and carries it to the ureter.
- The tissue of a kidney is composed of masses of tiny tubes called **kidney tubules** or **nephrons**. These are the structures that make the urine.
- High-pressure blood is supplied to the nephron via a tuft of capillaries called the **glomerulus**. Most of the contents of the blood except the cells and large protein molecules filter from the glomerulus into the (**Bowmans**) **capsule.** This fluid flows down a coiled part of the tubule (**proximal convoluted tubule**) where useful substances like glucose, amino acids and various ions are reabsorbed. The fluid flows to a looped portion of the tubule called the **Loop of Henle** where water is reabsorbed and then to another coiled part of the tubule (**distal convoluted tubule**) where more reabsorbtion and secretion takes place. Finally the fluid passes down the **collecting duct** where water is reabsorbed to form concentrated urine.

Worksheet

Use this Excretory System Worksheet [2] to help you learn the parts of the urinary system, the kidney and kidney tubule and their functions.

Test Yourself

The Urinary System Test Yourself can then be used to see if you understand this rather complex system.

1. Add the following labels to the diagram of the excretory system shown below. Bladder I ureter I urethra I kidney I dorsal aorta I vena cava I renal artery I vein

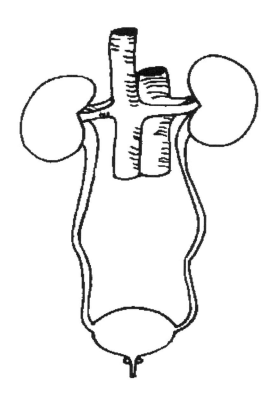

2. Using the words/phrases in the list below fill in the blanks in the following statements.

I cortex I amino acids I renal I glucose I water reabsorption I large proteins I

I bowman's capsule I diabetes mellitus I secreted I antidiuretic hormone (ADH) I blood cells I

I glomerulus I concentration of the urine I medulla I nephron I

a) Blood enters the kidney via the .... artery.

b) When cut across the kidney is seen to consist of two regions, the outer.............. and the inner..............

c) Another word for the kidney tubule is the...............................

d) Filtration of the blood occurs in the..............................

e) The filtered fluid (filtrate) enters the.............................

f) The filtrate entering the e) above is similar to blood but does not contain.................. or....................

g) As the fluid passes along the first coiled part of the kidney tubule.................. and.................... are removed.

h) The main function of the loop of Henle is..

i) Hydrogen and potassium ions are.............................. into the second coiled part of the tubule.

j) The main function of the collecting tube is..

k) The hormone...................................... is responsible for controlling water reabsorption in the collecting tube.

l) When the pancreas secretes inadequate amounts of the hormone insulin the condition known as..............................
results. This is most easily diagnosed by testing for................................ in the urine.

Test Yourself Answers

Websites

- http://www.biologycorner.com/bio3/nephron.html Biology Corner. A fabulous drawing of the kidney and nephron to print off, label and colour in with clear explanation of function.
- http://health.howstuffworks.com/adam-200032.htm How Stuff Works. This animation traces the full process of urine formation and reabsorption in the kidneys, its path down the ureter to the bladder, and its excretion via the urethra. Needs Shockwave.
- http://en.wikipedia.org/wiki/Nephron Wikipedia. A bit more detail than you need but still good clear explanations and lots of information.

Glossary

- Link to Glossary [4]

References

[1] http://flickr.com/photos/fazen/2615416/
[2] http://www.wikieducator.org/Excretory_System_Worksheet

Anatomy and Physiology of Animals/Urinary System/Test Yourself Answers

1. Add the following labels to the diagram of the excretory system shown below. Bladder | ureter | urethra | kidney | dorsal aorta | vena cava | renal artery | vein

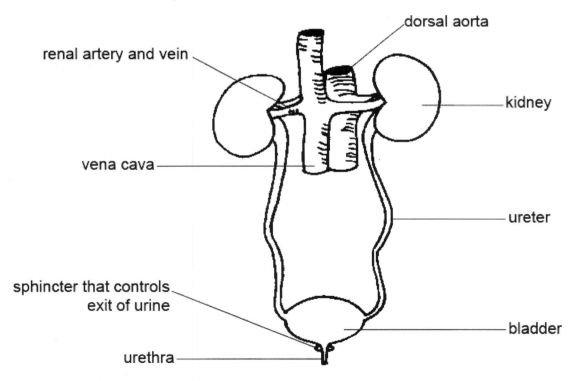

2. Fill in the blanks in the following statements.

a) Blood enters the kidney via the *renal artery*.

b) When cut across the kidney is seen to consist of two regions, the outer *cortex* and the inner *medulla*.

c) Another word for the kidney tubule is the *nephron*.

d) Filtration of the blood occurs in the *glomerulus*.

e) The filtered fluid (filtrate) enters the *Bowman's capsule*.

f) The filtrate entering the e) above is similar to blood but does not contain *large proteins* or *blood cells*.

g) As the fluid passes along the first coiled part of the kidney tubule *amino acids* and *glucose* are removed.

h) The main function of the loop of Henle is *water re-absorption/concentration of urine*.

i) Hydrogen and potassium ions are *secreted* into the second coiled part of the tubule.

j) The main function of the collecting tube is *concentration* of the urine.

k) The hormone *antidiuretic hormone (ADH)* is responsible for controlling the concentration of urine in the collecting tube.

l) When the pancreas secretes inadequate amounts of the hormone insulin the condition known as *diabetes mellitus* results. This is most easily diagnosed by testing for *glucose* in the urine.

Anatomy and Physiology of Animals/Reproductive System

Objectives

After completing this section, you should know:

- the role of mitosis and meiosis in the production of gametes (sperm and ova)
- that gametes are haploid cells
- that fertilization forms a diploid zygote
- the major parts of the male reproductive system and their functions
- the route sperm travel along the male reproductive tract to reach the penis
- the structure of a sperm and the difference between sperm and semen
- the difference between infertility and impotence
- the main parts of the female reproductive system and their functions
- the ovarian cycle and the roles of FSH, LH, oestrogen and progesterone
- the oestrous cycle and the signs of heat in rodents, dogs, cats and cattle
- the process of fertilization and where it occurs in the female tract
- what a morula and a blastocyst are
- what the placenta is and its functions

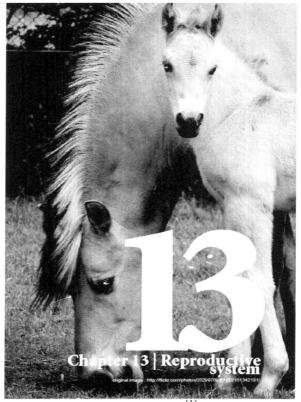

Chapter 13 | Reproductive system

original image by ynskjen [1] cc by

Reproductive System

In biological terms sexual reproduction involves the union of **gametes** - the sperm and the ovum - produced by two parents. Each gamete is formed by **meiosis** (see Chapter 3). This means each contains only half the chromosomes of the body cells (**haploid**). Fertilization results in the joining of the male and female gametes to form a **zygote** which contains the full number of chromosomes (**diploid**). The zygote then starts to divide by **mitosis** (see Chapter 3) to form a new animal with all its body cells containing chromosomes that are identical to those of the original zygote (see diagram 13.1).

Diagram 13.1 - Sexual reproduction

The offspring formed by sexual reproduction contain genes from both parents and show considerable variation. For example, kittens in a litter are all different although they (usually) have the same mother and father. In the wild this variation is important because it means that when the environment changes some individuals may be better adapted to survive than others. These survivors pass their "superior" genes on to their offspring. In this way the characteristics of a group of animals can gradually change over time to keep pace with the changing environment. This "survival of the fittest" or "**natural selection**" is the mechanism behind the theory of **evolution**.

Fertilisation

In most fish and amphibia (frogs and toads) fertilisation of the egg cells takes place outside the body. The female lays the eggs and then the male deposits his sperm on or at least near them.

In reptiles and birds, eggs are fertilized inside the body when the male deposits the sperm inside the **egg duct** of the female. The egg is then surrounded by a resistant shell, "laid" by the female and the embryo completes its development inside the egg.

In mammals the sperm are placed in the body of the female and the eggs are fertilized internally. They then develop to quite an advanced stage inside the body of the female. When they are born they are fed on milk excreted from the mammary glands and protected by their parents until they become independent.

Sexual Reproduction In Mammals

The reproductive organs of mammals produce the **gametes** (sperm and egg cells), help them fertilise and then support the developing embryo.

The Male Reproductive System

The male reproductive system consists of a pair of testes that produce **sperm** (or **spermatozoa**), ducts that transport the sperm to the penis and glands that add secretions to the sperm to make **semen** (see diagram 13.2).

The various parts of the male reproductive system with a summary of their functions are shown in diagram 13.3.

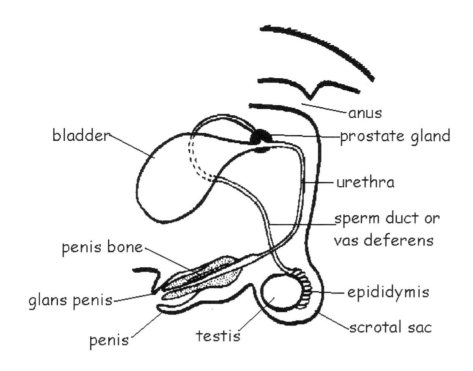

Diagram 13.2. The reproductive organs of a male dog

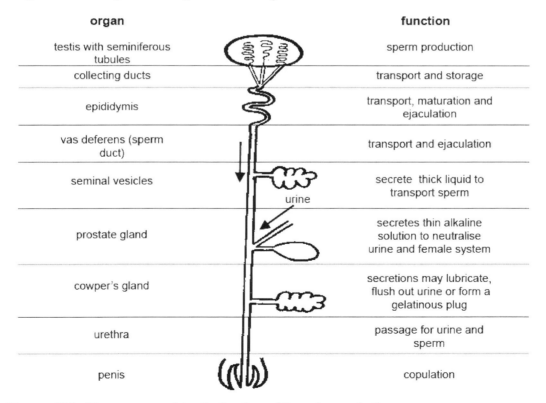

Diagram 13.3 - Diagram summarising the functions of the male reproductive organs

The Testes

Sperm need temperatures between 2 to 10 degrees Centigrade lower and then the body temperature to develop. This is the reason why the testes are located in a bag of skin called the **scrotal sacs** (or **scrotum**) that hangs below the body and where the evaporation of secretions from special glands can further reduce the temperature. In many animals (including humans) the testes descend into the scrotal sacs at birth but in some animals they do not descend until sexual maturity and in others they only descend temporarily during the breeding season. A mature animal in which one or both testes have not descended is called a **cryptorchid** and is usually infertile.

The problem of keeping sperm at a low enough temperature is even greater in birds that have a higher body temperature than mammals. For this reason bird's sperm are usually produced at night when the body temperature is lower and the sperm themselves are more resistant to heat.

The testes consist of a mass of coiled tubes (the **seminiferous** or **sperm producing tubules**) in which the sperm are formed by meiosis (see diagram 13.4). Cells lying between the seminiferous tubules produce the male sex hormone **testosterone**.

When the sperm are mature they accumulate in the **collecting ducts** and then pass to the **epididymis**before moving to the **sperm duct** or **vas deferens**. The two sperm ducts join the **urethra** just below the bladder, which passes through the **penis** and transports both sperm and urine.

Ejaculation discharges the semen from the erect penis. It is brought about by the contraction of the epididymis, vas deferens, prostate gland and urethra.

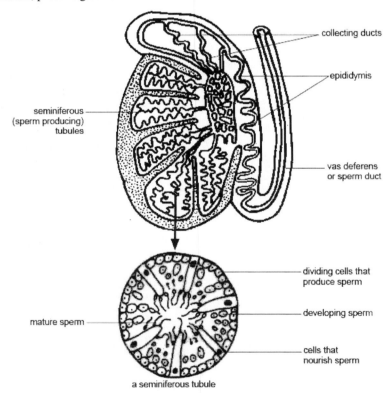

Diagram 13.4 - The testis and a magnified seminiferous tubule

Semen

Semen consists of 10% sperm and 90% fluid and as sperm pass down the ducts from testis to penis, (accessory) glands add various secretion

Accessory Glands

Three different glands may be involved in producing the secretions in which sperm are suspended, although the number and type of glands varies from species to species.

Seminal vesicles are important in rats, bulls, boars and stallions but are absent in cats and dogs. When present they produce secretions that make up much of the volume of the semen, and transport and provide nutrients for the sperm.

The **prostate gland** is important in dogs and humans. It produces an alkaline secretion that neutralizes the acidity of the male urethra and female vagina.

Cowper's glands have various functions in different species. The secretions may lubricate, flush out urine or form a gelatinous plug that traps the semen in the female reproductive system after copulation and prevents other males of the same species fertilizing an already mated female. Cowper's glands are absent in bears, dogs, and aquatic mammals.

The Penis

The penis consists of connective tissue with numerous small blood spaces in it. These fill with blood during sexual excitement causing erection.

Penis Form And Shape

Dogs, bears, seals, bats and rodents have a special bone in the penis which helps maintain the erection (see diagram 13.2). In some animals (e.g. the bull, ram and boar) the penis has an "S" shaped bend that allows it to fold up when not in use. In many animals the shape of the penis is adapted to match that of the vagina. For example, the boar has a corkscrew shaped penis, there is a pronounced twist in bulls' and it is forked in marsupials like the opossum. Some have spines, warts or hooks on them to help keep them in the vagina and copulation may be extended to help retain the semen in the female system. Mating can last up to three hours in minks, and dogs may "knot" or "tie" during mating and can not separate until the erection has subsided.

Sperm

Sperm are made up of three parts: a **head** consisting mainly of the nucleus, a **midpiece** containing many mitochondria to provide the energy and a **tail** that provides propulsion (see diagram 13.5).

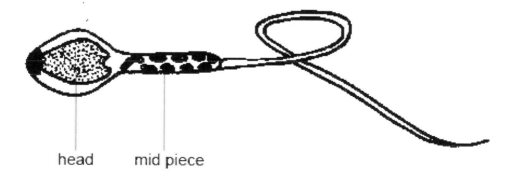

head   mid piece

Diagram 13.5 - A sperm

A single ejaculation may contain 2-3 hundred million sperm but even in normal semen as many as 10% of these sperm may be abnormal and infertile. Some may be dead while others are inactive or deformed with double, giant or small heads or tails that are coiled or absent altogether.

When there are too many abnormal sperm or when the sperm concentration is low, the semen may not be able to fertilize an egg and the animal is infertile. Make sure you don't confuse infertility with impotence, which is the inability to copulate successfully.

Sperm do not live forever. They have a definite life span that varies from species to species. They survive for between 20 days (guinea pig) to 60 days (bull) in the epididymis but once ejaculated into the female tract they only live from 12 to 48 hours. When semen is used for artificial insemination, storage under the right conditions can extend the life span of some species.

Artificial Insemination

In many species the male can be artificially stimulated to ejaculate and the semen collected. It can then be diluted, stored and used to **inseminate** females. For example bull semen can be diluted and stored for up to 3 weeks at room temperature. If mixed with an antifreeze solution and stored in "straws" in liquid nitrogen at minus 79°C it will keep for much longer. Unfortunately the semen of chickens, stallions and boars can only be stored for up to 2 days.

Dilution of the semen means that one male can be used to fertilise many more females than would occur under natural conditions. There are also advantages in the male and female not having to make physical contact. It means that owners of females do not have to buy expensive males and the possibility of transmitting sexually transmitted diseases is reduced. Routine examination of the semen for sperm concentration, quality and activity allows only the highest quality semen to be used so a high success rate is ensured.

Since the lifespan of sperm in the female tract is so short and ova only survive from 8 to 10 hours the timing of the artificial insemination is critical. Successful conception depends upon detecting the time that the animal is "on heat" and when ovulation occurs.

The Female Reproductive Organs

The female reproductive system consists of a pair of **ovaries** that produce egg cells or **ova** and **fallopian tubes** where fertilisation occurs and which carry the fertilised ovum to the **uterus**. Growth of the foetus takes place here. The **cervix** separates the uterus from the **vagina** or birth canal, where the sperm are deposited (see diagram 13.6).

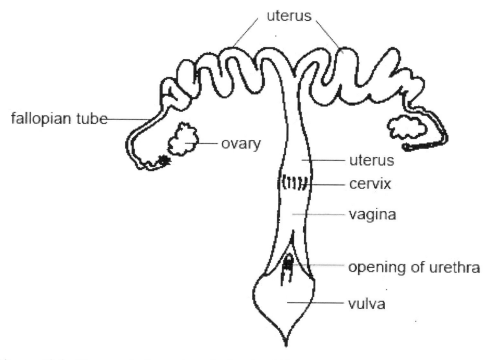

Diagram 13.6. - The reproductive system of a female rabbit

Note that primates like humans have a uterus with a single compartment but in most mammals the uterus is divided into two separate parts or **horns** as shown in diagram 13.6.

The Ovaries

Ovaries are small oval organs situated in the abdominal cavity just ventral to the kidneys. Most animals have a pair of ovaries but in birds only the left one is functional to reduce weight (see below).

The ovary consists of an inner region (**medulla**) and an outer region (**cortex**) containing egg cells or ova. These are formed in large numbers around the time of birth and start to develop after the animal becomes sexually mature. A cluster of cells called the **follicle** surrounds and nourishes each ovum.

The Ovarian Cycle

The **ovarian cycle** refers to the series of changes in the ovary during which the follicle matures, the ovum is shed and the **corpus luteum** develops (see diagram 13.7).

Numerous undeveloped ovarian follicles are present at birth but they start to mature after sexual maturity. In animals that normally have only one baby at a time only one ovum will mature at once but in litter animals several will. The mature follicle consists of outer cells that provide nourishment. Inside this is a fluid-filled space that contains the ovum.

A mature follicle can be quite large, ranging from a few millimetres in small mammals to the size of a golf ball in large animals. It bulges out from the surface of the ovary before eventually rupturing to release the ovum into the abdominal cavity. Once the ovum has been shed, a blood clot forms in the empty follicle. This develops into a tissue called the **corpus luteum** that produces the hormone **progesterone** (see diagram 13.9). If the animal becomes pregnant the corpus luteum persists, but if there is no pregnancy it degenerates and a new ovarian cycle usually.

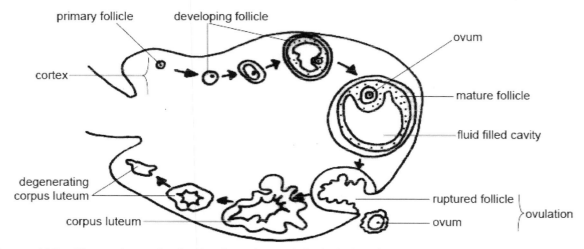

Diagram 13.7 - The ovarian cycle showing from the top left clockwise: the maturation of the ovum over time, followed by ovulation and the development of the corpus luteum in the empty follicle

The Ovum

When the ovum is shed the nucleus is in the final stages of meiosis (cell division). It is surrounded by several layers of follicle cells and a tough membrane called the **zona pelluc**ida (see diagram 13.8).

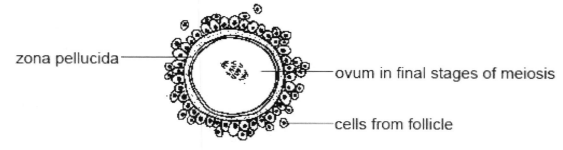

Diagram 13.8 - An ovum

The Oestrous Cycle

The **oestrous cycle** is the sequence of hormonal changes that occurs through the **ovarian cycle**. These changes influence the behaviour and body changes of the female (see diagram 13.9).

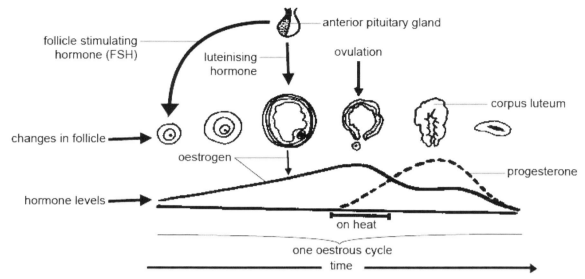

Diagram 13.9 - The oestrous cycle

The first hormone involved in the oestrous cycle is **follicle stimulating hormone (F.S.H.),** secreted by the **anterior pituitary gland** (see chapter 16). It stimulates the follicle to develop. As the follicle matures the outer cells begin to secrete the hormone **oestrogen** and this stimulates the mammary glands to develop. It also prepares the lining of the uterus to receive a fertilised egg. Ovulation is initiated by a surge of another hormone from the anterior pituitary, **luteinising hormone (L.H.).** This hormone also influences the development of the corpus luteum, which produces **progesterone**, a hormone that prepares the lining of the uterus for the fertilised ovum and readies the mammary glands for milk production. If no pregnancy takes place the corpus luteum shrinks and the production of progesterone decreases. This causes FSH to be produced again and a new oestrous cycle begins.

For fertilisation of the ovum by the sperm to occur, the female must be receptive to the male at around the time of ovulation. This is when the hormones turn on the signs of "**heat**", and she is "**in season**" or "**in oestrous**". These signs are turned off again at the end of the oestrous cycle.

During the oestrous cycle the lining of the uterus (**endometrium**) thickens ready for the fertilised ovum to be implanted. If no pregnancy occurs this thickened tissue is absorbed and the next cycle starts. In humans and other higher primates, however, the endometrium is shed as a flow of blood and instead of an oestrous cycle there is a **menstrual cycle**.

The length of the oestrous cycle varies from species to species. In rats the cycle only lasts 4-5 days and they are sexually receptive for about 14 hours. Dogs have a cycle that lasts 60-70 days and heat lasts 7-9 days and horses have a 21-day cycle and heat lasts an average of 6 days.

Ovulation is spontaneous in most animals but in some, e.g. the cat, and the rabbit, ovulation is stimulated by mating. This is called **induced ovulation**.

Signs Of Oestrous Or Heat

- When on heat a bitch has a blood stained discharge from the **vulva** that changes a little later to a straw coloured one that attracts all the dogs in the neighbourhood.
- Female cats "call" at night, roll and tread the carpet and are generally restless but will "stand" firm when pressure is placed on the pelvic region (this is the lordosis response).
- A female rat shows the lordosis response when on heat. It will "mount" other females and be more active than normal.
- A cow mounts other cows (bulling), bellows, is restless and has a discharge from the vulva.

Breeding Seasons And Breeding Cycles

Only a few animals breed throughout the year. This includes the higher primates (humans, gorillas and chimpanzees etc.), pigs, mice and rabbits. These are known as **continuous breeders**.

Most other animals restrict reproduction to one or two seasons in the year-**seasonal breeders** (see diagram 13.10). There are several reasons for this. It means the young can be born at the time (usually spring) when feed is most abundant and temperatures are favourable. It is also sensible to restrict the breeding season because courtship, mating, gestation and the rearing of young can exhaust the energy resources of an animal as well as make them more vulnerable to predators.

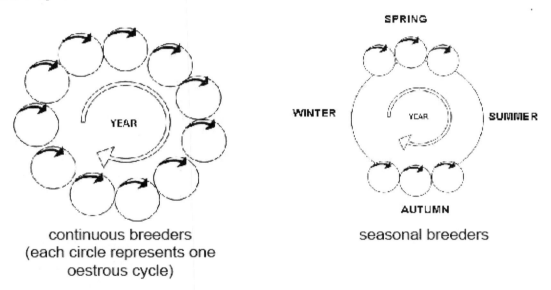

continuous breeders
(each circle represents one
oestrous cycle)

seasonal breeders

Diagram 13.10 - Breeding cycles

The timing of the breeding cycle is often determined by day length. For example the shortening day length in autumn will bring sheep and cows into season so the foetus can gestate through the winter and be born in spring. In cats the increasing day length after the winter solstice (shortest day) stimulates breeding. The number of times an animal comes into season during the year varies, as does the number of oestrous cycles during each season. For example a dog usually has 2-3 seasons per year, each usually consisting of just one oestrous cycle. In contrast ewes usually restrict breeding to one season and can continue to cycle as many as 20 times if they fail to become pregnant.

Fertilisation and Implantation

Fertilisation

The opening of the fallopian tube lies close to the ovary and after ovulation the ovum is swept into its funnel-like opening and is moved along it by the action of cilia and wave-like contractions of the wall.

Copulation deposits several hundred million sperm in the vagina. They swim through the cervix and uterus to the fallopian tubes moved along by whip-like movements of their tails and contractions of the uterus. During this journey the sperm undergo their final phase of maturation so they are ready to fertilise the ovum by the time they reach it in the upper fallopian tube.

High mortality means only a small proportion of those deposited actually reach the ovum. The sperm attach to the outer zona pellucida and enzymes secreted from a gland in the head of the sperm dissolve this membrane so it can enter. Once one sperm has entered, changes in the **zona pellucida** prevent further sperm from penetrating. The sperm loses its tail and the two nuclei fuse to form a **zygote** with the full set of paired chromosomes restored.

Development Of The Morula And Blastocyst

As the fertilised egg travels down the fallopian tube it starts to divide by mitosis. First two cells are formed and then four, eight, sixteen, etc. until there is a solid ball of cells. This is called a **morula**. As division continues a hollow ball of cells develops. This is a **blastocyst** (see diagram 13.11).

Implantation

Implantation involves the blastocyst attaching to, and in some species, completely sinking into the wall of the uterus.

Pregnancy

The Placenta And Foetal Membranes

As the **embryo** increases in size, the **placenta**, **umbilical cord** and **foetal membranes** (often known collectively as the **placenta**) develop to provide it with nutrients and remove waste products (see diagram 13.12). In later stages of development the embryo becomes known as a **foetus**.

The placenta is the organ that attaches the foetus to the wall of the uterus. In it the blood of the foetus and mother flow close to each other but never mix (see diagram 13.13). The closeness of the maternal and foetal blood systems allows diffusion between them. Oxygen and nutrients diffuse from the mother's blood into that of the foetus and carbon dioxide and excretory products diffuse in the other direction. Most maternal hormones (except adrenaline), antibodies, almost all drugs (including alcohol), lead and DDT also pass across the placenta. However, it protects the foetus from infection with bacteria and most viruses.

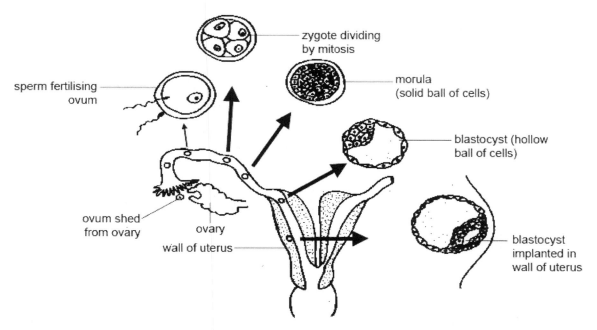

Diagram 13.11 - Development and implantation of the embryo

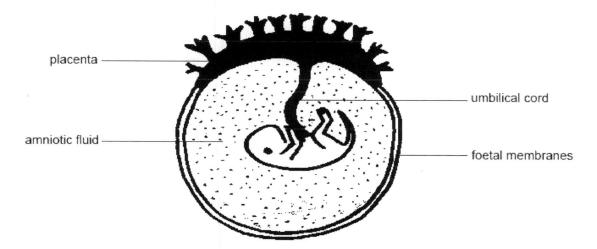

Diagram 13.12. The foetus and placenta

The foetus is attached to the placenta by the **umbilical cord**. It contains arteries that carry blood to the placenta and a vein that returns blood to the foetus. The developing foetus becomes surrounded by membranes. These enclose the amniotic fluid that protects the foetus from knocks and other trauma (see diagram 13.12).

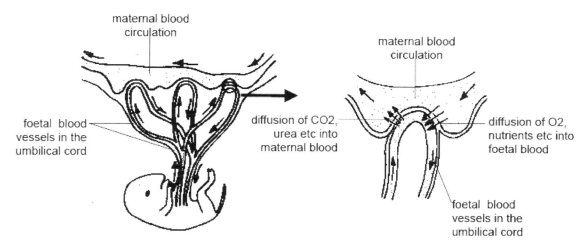

Diagram 13.13 - Maternal and foetal blood flow in the placenta

Hormones During Pregnancy

The corpus luteum continues to secrete progesterone and oestrogen during pregnancy. These maintain the lining of the uterus and prepare the mammary glands for milk secretion. Later in the pregnancy the placenta itself takes over the secretion of these hormones.

Chorionic gonadotrophin is another hormone secreted by the placenta and placental membranes. It prevents uterine contractions before labour and prepares the mammary glands for lactation. Towards the end of pregnancy the placenta and ovaries secrete **relaxin**, a hormone that eases the joint between the two parts of the pelvis and helps dilate the cervix ready for birth.

Pregnancy Testing

The easiest method of pregnancy detection is ultrasound which is noninvasive and very reliable Later in gestation pregnancy can be detected by taking x-rays.

In dogs and cats a blood test can be used to detect the hormone **relaxin**.

In mares and cows palpation of the uterus via the rectum is the classic way to determine pregnancy. It can also be done by detecting the hormones **progesterone** or **equine chorionic gonagotrophin** (**eCG**) in the urine. A new sensitive test measures the amount of the hormone, **oestrone sulphate**, present in a sample of faeces. The hormone is produced by the foal and placenta, and is only present when there is a living foal.

In most animals, once pregnancy is advanced, there is a window of time during which an experienced veterinarian can determine pregnancy by feeling the abdomen.

Gestation Period

The young of many animals (e.g. pigs, horses and elephants) are born at an advanced state of development, able to stand and even run to escape predators soon after they are born. These animals have a relatively long gestation period that varies with their size e.g. from 114 days in the pig to 640 days in the elephant.

In contrast, cats, dogs, mice, rabbits and higher primates are relatively immature when born and totally dependent on their parents for survival. Their gestation period is shorter and varies from 25 days in the mouse to 31 days in rabbits and 258 days in the gorilla.

The babies of marsupials are born at an extremely immature stage and migrate to the pouch where they attach to a teat to complete their development. Kangaroo joeys, for example, are born 33 days after conception and opossums after only 8 days.

Birth

Signs Of Imminent Birth

As the pregnancy continues, the mammary glands enlarge and may secrete a milky substance a few days before birth occurs. The vulva may swell and produce thick mucus and there is sometimes a visible change in the position of the foetus. Just before birth the mother often becomes restless, lying down and getting up frequently. Many animals seek a secluded place where they may build a nest in which to give birth.

Labour

Labour involves waves of uterine contractions that press the foetus against the cervix causing it to dilate. The foetus is then pushed through the cervix and along the vagina before being delivered. In the final stage of labour the placenta or "afterbirth" is expelled.

Adaptations Of The Foetus To Life Outside The Uterus

The foetus grows in the watery, protected environment of the uterus where the mother supplies oxygen and nutrients, and waste products pass to her blood circulation for excretion. Once the baby animal is born it must start to breathe for itself, digest food and excrete its own waste. To allow these functions to occur blood is re-routed to the lungs and the glands associated with the gut start to secrete. Note that newborn animals can not control their own body temperature. They need to be kept warm by the mother, littermates and insulating nest materials.

Milk Production

Cows, manatees and primates have two mammary glands but animals like pigs that give birth to large litters may have as many as 12 pairs. Ducts from the gland lead to a nipple or teat and there may be a sinus where the milk collects before being suckled (see diagram 13.14).

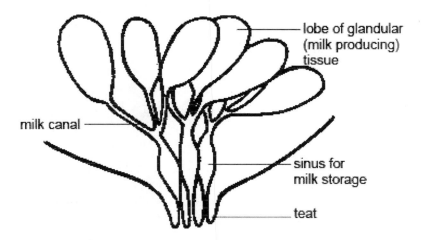

Diagram 13.14 - A mammary gland

The hormones **oestrogen** and **progesterone** stimulate the mammary glands to develop and **prolactin** promotes the secretion of the milk. **Oxytocin** from the pituitary gland releases the milk when the baby suckles. The first milk is called **colostrum**. It is a rich in nutrients and contains protective antibodies from the mother. Milk contains fat, protein and milk sugar as well as vitamins and most minerals although it contains little iron. Its actual composition varies widely from species to species. For example whale's and seal's milk has twelve times more fat and four times more protein than cow's milk. Cow's milk has far less protein in it than cat's or dog's milk. This is why orphan kittens and puppies cannot be fed cow's milk.

Reproduction In Birds

Male birds have testes and sperm ducts and male swans, ducks, geese and ostriches have a penis. However, most birds make do with a small amount of erectile tissue known as a **papilla**. To reduce weight for flight most female birds only have one ovary - usually the left, which produces extremely yolky eggs. The eggs are fertilised in the upper part of the oviduct (equivalent to the fallopian tube and uterus of mammals) and as they pass down it **albumin** (the white of the egg), the membrane beneath the shell and the shell are laid down over the yolk. Finally the egg is covered in a layer of mucus to help the bird lay it (see diagram 13.15).

Most birds lay their eggs in a nest and the hen sits on them until they hatch. Ducklings and chicks are relatively well developed when they hatch and able to forage for their own food. Most other nestlings need their parents to keep them warm, clean and fed. Young birds grow rapidly and have voracious appetites that may involve the parents making up to 1000 trips a day to supply their need for food.

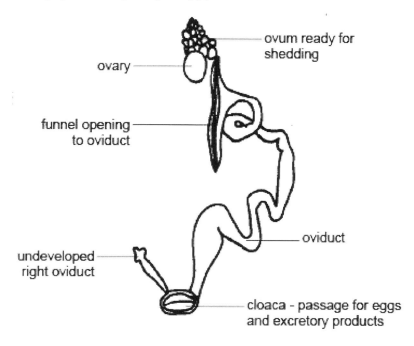

Diagram 13.15 - Female reproductive organs of a bird

Summary

- **Haploid** gametes (sperm and ova) are produced by meiosis in the **gonads** (testes and ovaries).
- Fertilisation involves the fusing of the gametes to form a diploid **zygote**.
- The male reproductive system consists of a pair of **testes** that produce sperm (or **spermatozoa**), ducts that transport the sperm to the penis and glands that add secretions to the sperm to make semen.
- Sperm are produced in the **seminiferous tubules**, are stored in the **epididymis** and travel via the **vas deferens** or **sperm duct** to the junction of the bladder and the **urethra** where various accessory glands add secretions. The fluid is now called **semen** and is ejaculated into the female system down the **urethra** that runs down the centre of the penis.
- Sperm consist of a head, a midpiece and a tail.
- **Infertility** is the inability of sperm to fertilize an egg while **impotence** is the inability to copulate successfully.
- The female reproductive system consists of a pair of **ovaries** that produce **ova** and **fallopian tubes** where fertilisation occurs and which carry the fertilised ovum to the **uterus**. Growth of the foetus takes place here. The **cervix** separates the uterus from the **vagina**, the birth canal and where the sperm are deposited.

- The **ovarian cycle** refers to the series of changes in the ovary during which the follicle matures, the ovum is shed and the **corpus luteum** develops.

- The **oestrous cycle** is the sequence of hormonal changes that occurs through the ovarian cycle. It is initiated by the secretion of **follicle stimulating hormone (F.S.H.),** by the **anterior pituitary gland** which stimulates the **follicle** to develop. The follicle secretes **oestrogen** which stimulates **mammary gland** development. **luteinising hormone (L.H.)** from the anterior pituitary initiates **ovulation** and stimulates the **corpus luteum** to develop. The corpus luteum produces **progesterone** that prepares the lining of the uterus for the fertilised ovum.

- **Signs of oestrous** or heat differ. A bitch has a blood stained discharge, female cats and rats are restless and show the lordosis response, while cows mount other cows, bellow and have a discharge from the vulva.

- After fertilisation in the fallopian tube the **zygote** divides over and over by mitosis to become a ball of cells called a **morula**. Division continues to form a hollow ball of cells called the **blastocyst**. This is the stage that **implants** in the uterus.

- The **placenta, umbilical cord** and **foetal membranes** (known as the **placenta**) protect and provide the developing foetus with nutrients and remove waste products.

Worksheet

Reproductive System Worksheet [2]

Test Yourself

1. Add the following labels to the diagram of the male reproductive organs below.

> testis | epididymis | vas deferens | urethra | penis | scrotal sac | prostate gland

Diagram of the Male Reproductive System

2. Match the following descriptions with the choices given in the list below.

> accessory glands | vas deferens or sperm duct | penis | scrotum | fallopian tube | testes | urethra | vagina | uterus | ovary | vulva

a) Organ that delivers semen to the female vagina

b) Where the sperm are produced

c) Passage for sperm from the epididymis to the urethra

d) Carries both sperm and urine down the penis

e) Glands that produce secretions that make up most of the semen

f) Bag of skin surrounding the testes

g) Where the foetus develops

h) This receives the penis during copulation

i) Where fertilisation usually occurs

j) Ova travel along this tube to reach the uterus

k) Where the ova are produced

l) The external opening of the vagina

3. Which hormone is described in each statement below?

a) This hormone stimulates the growth of the follicles in the ovary

b) This hormone converts the empty follicle into the corpus luteum and stimulates it to produce progesterone

c) This hormone is produced by the cells of the follicle

d) This hormone is produced by the corpus luteum

   e) This hormone causes the mammary glands to develop

   f) This hormone prepares the lining of the uterus to receive a fertilised ovum

4. State whether the following statements are true or false. If false write in the correct answer.

   a) Fertilisation of the egg occurs in the uterus

   b) The fertilised egg cell contains half the normal number of chromosomes

   c) The morula is a hollow ball of cells

   d) The mixing of the blood of the mother and foetus allows nutrients and oxygen to transfer easily to the foetus

   e) The morula implants in the wall of the uterus

   f) The placenta is the organ that supplies the foetus with oxygen and nutrients

   g) Colostrum is the first milk

   h) Young animals often have to be given calcium supplements because milk contains very little calcium

Test Yourself Answers

Websites

- http://www.anatomicaltravel.com/CB_site/Conception_to_birth3.htm Anatomical travel. Images of fertilisation and the development of the (human) embryo through to birth.

- http://www.uchsc.edu/ltc/fert.swf Fertilisation. A great animation of fertilisation, formation of the zygote and first mitotic division. A bit advanced but still worth watching.

- http://www.uclan.ac.uk/facs/health/nursing/sonic/scenarios/salfordanim/heart.swf Sonic. An animation showing the foetal blood circulation through the placenta to the changes allowing circulation through the lungs after birth.

- http://en.wikipedia.org/wiki/Estrus Wikipedia. As always, good interesting information although some terms and concepts are beyond the requirements of this level.

Glossary

- Link to Glossary [4]

References

[1] http://flickr.com/photos/20299709@N00/151342191/
[2] http://www.wikieducator.org/Reproductive_System_Worksheet

Anatomy and Physiology of Animals/Reproductive System/Test Yourself Answers

1. Add the following labels to the diagram of the male reproductive organs below.

testis | epididymis | vas deferens | urethra | penis | scrotal sac | prostate gland

Diagram of Male Reproductive System with labels added

2. Match the following descriptions with the choices given in the list below.

accessory glands | vas deferens or sperm duct | penis | scrotum | fallopian tube | testes | urethra | vagina | uterus | ovary | vulva

a) The *penis* delivers semen to the female vagina.

b) The sperm are produced in the *testes*.

c) The *vas deferens* or *sperm duct* is the passage for sperm from the epididymis to the penis.

d) The *urethra* carries both sperm and urine down the penis.

e) *Accessory glands* produce secretions that make up most of the semen.

f) The *scrotum* is the bag of skin surrounding the testes.

g) The foetus develops in the *uterus*.

h) The *vagina* receives the penis during copulation.

i) Fertilisation usually occurs in the *fallopian tube*.

j) Ova travel along the *fallopian tube* to reach the uterus.

k) The ova are produced in the *ovary*.

l) The *vulva* is the external opening of the vagina.

3. Which hormone is described in each statement below?

a) *Follicle stimulating hormone (FSH)* stimulates the growth of the follicles in the ovary.

b) *Luteinising hormone (LH)* converts the empty follicle into the corpus luteum and stimulates it to produce progesterone.

c) *Oestrogen* is produced by the cells of the follicle.

d) *Progesterone* is produced by the corpus luteum.

e) *Oestrogen* causes the mammary glands to develop.

f) *Progesterone* prepares the lining of the uterus to receive a fertilised ovum.

4. State whether the following statements are true or false. If false write in the correct answer.

a) Fertilisation of the egg occurs in the uterus.

False - Fertilisation normally occurs in the fallopian tube.

b) The fertilised egg cell contains half the normal number of chromosomes.

False - Once fertilised the normal (diploid or 2n) number of chromosomes are restored.

c) The morula is a hollow ball of cells.

False - The morula is a solid ball of cells. It is the blastocyst that is hollow.

d) Mixing of the blood of the mother and foetus allows nutrients and oxygen to transfer easily to the foetus.

False - There is no mixing of foetal and maternal blood in the placenta.

e) The morula implants in the wall of the uterus.

False. It is the blastocyst that implants in the wall of the uterus.

f) The placenta is the organ that supplies the foetus with oxygen and nutrients.

True.

g) To adjust the baby animal to the outside world the blood has to be re-routed to the lungs.

True. In the uterus the foetal lungs are inactive and once the baby is born and starts to breathe blood has to be supplied to the lungs so it can be oxygenated.

h) Colostrum is the first milk.

True.

i) Young animals often have to be given calcium supplements because milk contains very little calcium.

False. Milk contains lots of calcium. What it lacks is iron and this often has to be given as a supplement.

Anatomy and Physiology of Animals/Nervous System

Objectives

After completing this section, you should know:

- the role of the nervous system in coordinating an animal's response to the environment
- that the nervous system gathers, sorts and stores information and initiates movement
- the basic structure and function of a neuron
- the structure and function of a synapse and neurotransmitter chemicals
- the nervous pathway known as a reflex with examples
- that training can develop conditioned reflexes in animals
- that the nervous system can be divided into the central and peripheral nervous systems
- that the brain is surrounded by membranes called meninges
- the basic parts of the brain and the function of the cerebral hemispheres, hypothalamus, pituitary, cerebellum and medulla oblongata
- the structure and function of the spinal cord
- that the peripheral nervous system consists of cranial and spinal nerves and the autonomic nervous system
- that the autonomic nervous system consists of sympathetic and parasympathetic parts with different functions

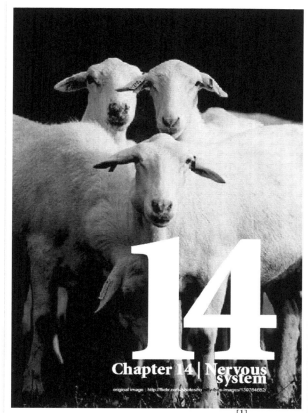

original image by Royalty-free image collection [1] cc by

Coordination

Animals must be able to sense and respond to the environment in which they live if they are to survive. They need to be able to sense the temperature of their surroundings, for example, so they can avoid the hot sun. They must also be able to identify food and escape predators.

The various systems and organs in the body must also be linked so they work together. For example, once a predator has identified suitable prey it has to catch it. This involves coordinating the contraction of the muscle so the predator can run, there must then be an increased blood supply to the muscles to provide them with oxygen and nutrients. At the same time the respiration rate must increase to supply the oxygen and remove the carbon dioxide produced as a result of this increased activity. Once the prey has been caught and eaten, the digestive system must be activated to digest it.

The adjustment of an animal's response to changes in the environment and the complex linking of the various processes in the body that this response involves are called **co-ordination**. Two systems are involved in co-ordination in animals. These are the **nervous** and **endocrine systems**. The first operates via electrical impulses along nerve fibres and the second by releasing special chemicals or hormones into the bloodstream from glands.

Functions of the Nervous System

The nervous system has three basic functions:

1. **Sensory function** - to sense changes (known as stimuli) both outside and within the body. For example the eyes sense changes in light and the ear responds to sound waves. Inside the body, tretch receptors in the stomach indicate when it is full and chemical receptors in the blood vessels monitor the acidity of the blood.

2. **Integrative function** - processing the information received from the sense organs. The impulses from these organs are analysed and stored as memory. The many different impulses from different sources are sorted, synchronised and co-ordinated and the appropriate response initiated. The power to integrate, remember and apply experience gives higher animals much of their superiority.

3. **Motor function** - The third function is the response to the stimuli that causes muscles to contract or glands to secrete.

All nervous tissue is made up of nerve cells or **neurons.** These transmit high-speed signals called **nerve impulses**. Nerve impulses can be thought of as being similar to an electric current.

The Neuron

Neurons are cells that have been adapted to carry nerve impulses. A typical neuron has a **cell body** containing a nucleus, one or more branching filaments called **dendrites** which conduct nerve impulses towards the cell body and one long fibre, an **axon**, that carries the impulses away from it. Many axons have a sheath of fatty material called **myelin** surrounding them. This speeds up the rate at which the nerve impulses travel along the nerve (see diagram 14.1).

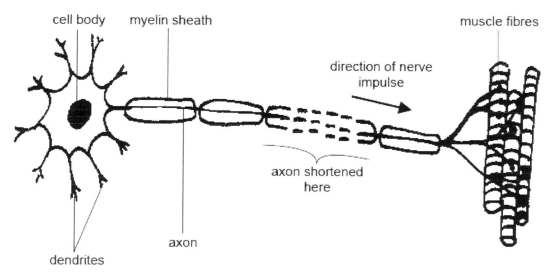

Diagram 14.1 - A motor neuron

The cell body of neurons is usually located in the brain or spinal cord while the axon extends the whole distance to the organ that it supplies. The neuron carrying impulses from the spinal cord to the hind leg or tail of a horse, for example, can be several feet long. A **nerve** is a bundle of axons.

A **sensory neuron** is a nerve cell that transmits impulses from a sense receptor such as those in the eye or ear to the brain or spinal cord. A **motor neuron** is a nerve cell that transmits impulses from the brain or spinal cord to a muscle or gland. A **relay neuron** connects sensory and motor neurons and is found in the brain or spinal cord (see diagrams 14.1 and 14.2).

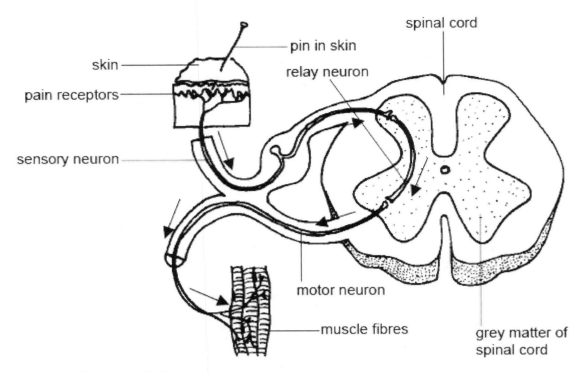

Diagram 14.2 - The relationship between sensory, relay and motor neurons

Connections Between Neurons

The connection between adjacent neurons is called a **synapse**. The two nerve cells do not actually touch here for there is a microscopic space between them. The electrical impulse in the neurone before the synapse stimulates the production of chemicals called **neurotransmitters** (such as **acetylcholine**), which are secreted into the gap.

The neurotransmitter chemicals diffuse across the gap and when they contact the membrane of the next nerve cell they stimulate a new nervous impulse (see diagram 14.3). After the impulse has passed the chemical is destroyed and the synapse is ready to receive the next nerve impulse.

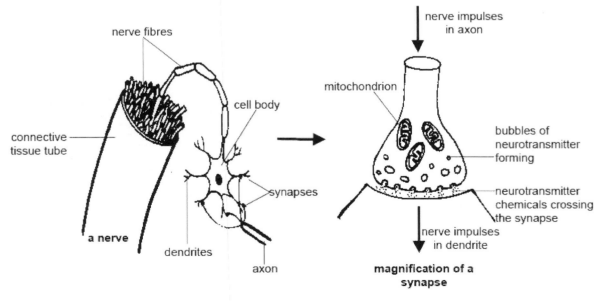

Diagram 14.3 - A nerve and magnification of a synapse

Reflexes

A **reflex** is a rapid automatic response to a stimulus. When you accidentally touch a hot object and automatically jerk your hand away, this is a reflex action. It happens without you having to think about it. Animals automatically blink when an object approaches the eye and cats twist their bodies in the air when falling so they land on their paws. (Please don't test this one at home with your pet cat!).

Swallowing, sneezing, and the constriction of the pupil of the eye in bright light are also all reflex actions.

The path taken by the nerve impulses in a reflex is called a **reflex arc**. Most reflex arcs involve only three neurons (see diagram 14.4). The **stimulus** (a pin in the paw) stimulates the pain receptors of the skin, which initiate an impulse in a sensory neuron. This travels to the spinal cord where it passes, by means of a synapse, to a connecting neuron called the relay neuron situated in the spinal cord. The relay neuron in turn makes a synapse with one or more motor neurons that transmit the impulse to the muscles of the limb causing them to contract and remove the paw from the sharp object. Reflexes do not require involvement of the brain although you are aware of what is happening and can, in some instances, prevent them happening. Animals are born with their reflexes. You can think of them as being wired in.

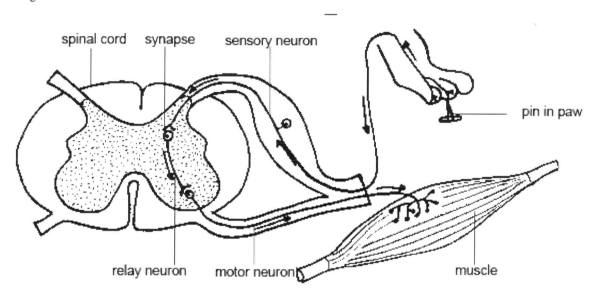

Diagram 14.4 - A reflex arc

Conditioned Reflexes

In most reflexes the stimulus and response are related. For example the presence of food in the mouth causes the salivary glands to release saliva. However, it is possible to train animals (and humans) to respond to different and often quite irrelevant stimuli. This is called a **conditioned reflex**.

A Russian biologist called Pavlov carried out the classic experiment to demonstrate such a reflex when he conditioned dogs to salivate at the sound of a bell ringing. Almost every pet owner can identify reflexes they have conditioned in their animals. Perhaps you have trained your cat to associate food with the opening of the fridge door or accustomed your dog to the routines you go through before taking them for a walk.

Parts of the Nervous System

When we describe the nervous system of vertebrates we usually divide it into two parts (see diagram 14.5).

    1. The **central nervous system** (**CNS**) which consists of the brain and spinal cord.

    2. The **peripheral nervous system** (**PNS**) which consists of the nerves that connect to the brain and spinal cord (cranial and spinal nerves) as well as the **autonomic** (or involuntary) nervous system.

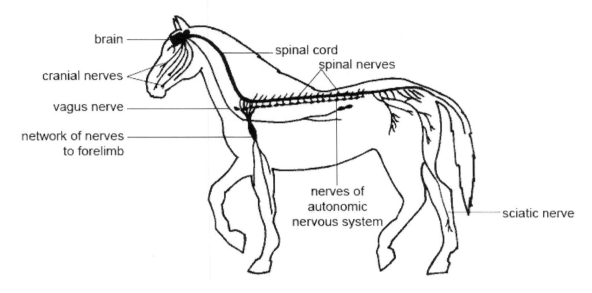

Diagram 14.5 - The nervous system of a horse

The Central Nervous System

The **central nervous system** consists of the brain and spinal cord. It acts as a kind of 'telephone exchange' where a vast number of cross connections are made.

When you look at the brain or spinal cord some regions appear creamy white (**white matter**) and others appear grey (**grey matter**). White matter consists of masses of nerve axons and the grey matter consists of the nerve cells. In the brain the grey matter is on the outside and in the spinal cord it is on the inside (see diagram 14.2).

The Brain

The major part of the brain lies protected within the sturdy "box" of skull called the **cranium**. Surrounding the fragile brain tissue (and spinal cord) are protective membranes called the **meninges** (see diagram 14.6), and a crystal-clear fluid called **cerebrospinal fluid**, which protects and nourishes the brain tissue. This fluid also fills four cavities or **ventricles** that lie within the brain.

Brain tissue is extremely active and, even when an animal is resting, it uses up to 20% of the oxygen taken into the body by the lungs. The **carotid artery**, a branch off the dorsal aorta, supplies it with the oxygen and nutrients it requires. Brain damage occurs if brain tissue is deprived of oxygen for only 4-8 minutes.

The brain consists of three major regions:

    1. the **fore brain** which includes the **cerebral hemispheres**, **hypothalamus** and **pituitary gland**;

    2. the **hind brain** or **brain stem**, contains the **medulla oblongata** and **pons** and

    3. the **cerebellum** or "little brain" (see diagram 14.6).

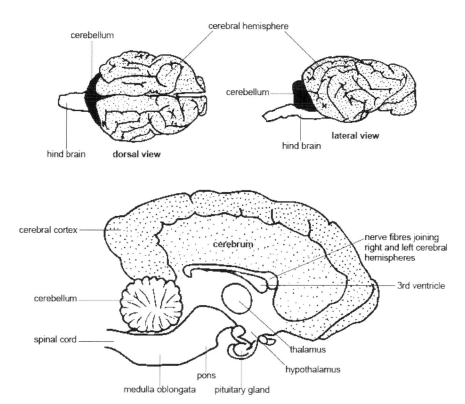

Diagram 14.6 - Longitudinal section through the brain of a dog

Mapping the brain

In humans and some animals the functions of the different regions of the cerebral cortex have been mapped (see diagram 14.7).

Diagram 14.7 - The functions of the regions of the human cerebral cortex

The Forebrain

The **cerebral hemispheres** are the masses of brain tissue that sit on the top of the brain. The surface is folded into ridges and furrows called **sulci** (singular sulcus). They make this part of the brain look rather like a very large walnut kernel. The two hemispheres are separated by a deep groove although they are connected internally by a thick bundle of nerve fibres. The outer layer of each hemisphere is called the **cerebral cortex** and this is where the main functions of the cerebral hemispheres are carried out.

The cerebral cortex is large and convoluted in mammals compared to other vertebrates and largest of all in humans because this is where the so-called "higher centres" concerned with memory, learning, reasoning and intelligence are situated.

Nerves from the eyes, ears, nose and skin bring sensory impulses to the cortex where they are interpreted. Appropriate voluntary movements are initiated here in the light of the memories of past events.

Different regions of the cortex are responsible for particular sensory and motor functions, e.g. vision, hearing, taste, smell, or moving the fore-limbs, hind-limbs or tail. For example, when a dog sniffs a scent, sensory impulses from the organ of smell in the nose pass via the olfactory (smelling) nerve to the olfactory centres of the cerebral hemispheres where the impulses are interpreted and co-ordinated.

In humans and some animals the functions of the different regions of the cerebral cortex have been mapped (see diagram 14.8).

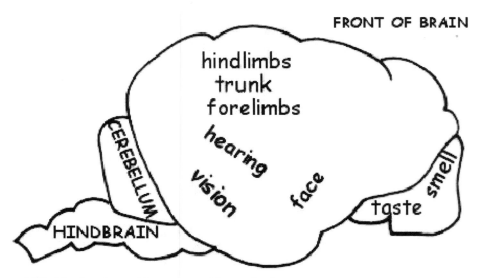

Diagram 14.8 - The functions of the regions of the cerebral cortex

The **hypothalamus** is situated at the base of the brain and is connected by a "stalk" to the **pituitary gland**, the "master" hormone-producing gland (see chapter 16). The hypothalamus can be thought of as the bridge between the nervous and endocrine (hormone producing) systems. It produces some of the hormones that are released from the pituitary gland and controls the release of others from it.

It is also an important centre for controlling the internal environment of the animal and therefore maintaining homeostasis. For example, it helps regulate the movement of food through the gut and the temperature, blood pressure and concentration of the blood. It is also responsible for the feeling of being hungry or thirsty and it controls sleep patterns and sex drive.

The Hindbrain

The **medulla oblongata** is at the base of the brain and is a continuation of the spinal cord. It carries all signals between the spinal cord and the brain and contains centres that control vital body functions like the basic rhythm of breathing, the rate of the heartbeat and the activities of the gut. The medulla oblongata also co-ordinates swallowing, vomiting, coughing and sneezing.

The Cerebellum

The **cerebellum** (little brain) looks rather like a smaller version of the cerebral hemispheres attached to the back of the brain. It receives impulses from the organ of balance (vestibular organ) in the inner ear and from stretch receptors in the muscles and tendons. By co-ordinating these it regulates muscle contraction during walking and running and helps maintain the posture and balance of the animal. When the cerebellum malfunctions it causes a tremor and uncoordinated movement.

The Spinal Cord

The spinal cord is a cable of nerve tissue that passes down the channel in the vertebrae from the hindbrain to the end of the tail. It becomes progressively smaller as paired **spinal nerves** pass out of the cord to parts of the body. Protective membranes or meninges cover the cord and these enclose cerebral spinal fluid (see diagram 14.9).

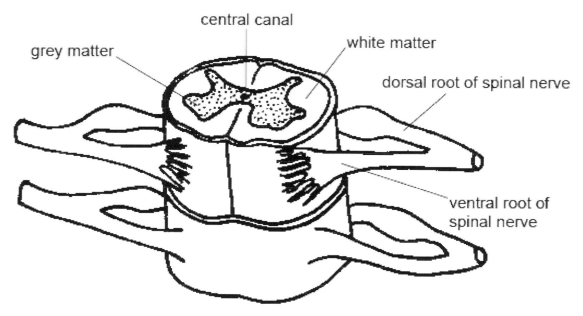

Diagram 14.9 - The spinal cord

If you cut across the spinal cord you can see that it consists of white matter on the outside and grey matter in the shape of an H or butterfly on the inside.

The Peripheral Nervous System

The **peripheral nervous system** consists of nerves that are connected to the brain (**cranial nerves**), and nerves that are connected to the spinal cord (**spinal nerves**). The **autonomic nervous** system **is also part of the peripheral nervous system.**

Cranial Nerves

There are twelve pairs of cranial nerves that come from the brain. Each passes through a hole in the cranium (brain case). The most important of these are the olfactory, optic, acoustic and vagus nerves.

The **olfactory nerves** - (smell) carry impulses from the olfactory organ of the nose to the brain.

The **optic nerves** - (sight) carry impulses from the retina of the eye to the brain.

The **auditory (acoustic) nerves** - (hearing) carry impulses from the cochlear of the inner ear to the brain.

The **vagus nerve** - controls the muscles that bring about swallowing. It also controls the muscles of the heart, airways, lungs, stomach and intestines (see diagram 14.5).

Spinal Nerves

Spinal nerves connect the spinal cord to sense organs, muscles and glands in the body. Pairs of spinal nerves leave the spinal cord and emerge between each pair of adjacent vertebrae (see diagram 14.9).

The **sciatic nerve** is the largest spinal nerve in the body (see diagram 14.5). It leaves the spinal cord as several nerves that join to form a flat band of nervous tissue. It passes down the thigh towards the hind leg where it gives off branches to the various muscles of this limb.

The Autonomic Nervous System

The **autonomic nervous system** controls internal body functions that are not under conscious control. For example when a prey animal is chased by a predator the autonomic nervous system automatically increases the rate of breathing and the heartbeat. It dilates the blood vessels that carry blood to the muscles, releases glucose from the liver, and makes other adjustments to provide for the sudden increase in activity. When the animal has escaped and is safe once again the nervous system slows down all these processes and resumes all the normal body activities like the digestion of food.

The nerves of the autonomic nervous system originate in the spinal cord and pass out between the vertebrae to serve the various organs (see diagram 14.10).There are two main parts to the autonomic nervous system -- the **sympathetic system** and the **parasympathetic system**.

The **sympathetic system** stimulates the "flight, fright, fight" response that allows an animal to face up to an attacker or make a rapid departure. It increases the heart and respiratory rates, as well as the amount of blood flowing to the skeletal muscles while blood flow to less critical regions like the gut and skin is reduced. It also causes the pupils of the eyes to dilate. Note that the effects of the sympathetic system are similar to the effects of the hormone adrenaline (see Chapter 16).

The **parasympathetic system** does the opposite to the sympathetic system. It maintains the normal functions of the relaxed body. These are sometimes known as the "housekeeping" functions. It promotes effective digestion, stimulates defaecation and urination and maintains a regular heartbeat and rate of breathing.

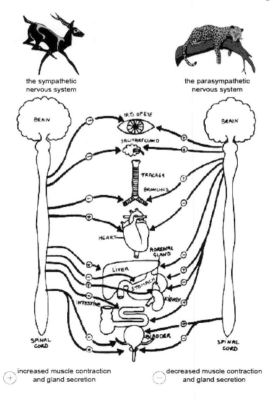

Diagram 14.10 - The function of the sympathetic and parasympathetic nervous systems

Summary

- The **neuron** is the basic unit of the nervous system. It consists of a **cell body** with a nucleus, filaments known as **dendrites** and a long fibre known as the **axon** often surrounded by a **myelin sheath**.
- A **nerve** is a bundle of axons.
- **Grey matter** in the brain and spinal cord consists mainly of brain ells while **white matter** consists of masses of axons.
- **Nerve Impulses** travel along axons.
- Adjacent neurons connect with each other at **synapses**.
- **Reflexes** are automatic responses to stimuli. The path taken by nerve impulses involved in reflexes is a **reflex arc**. Most reflex arcs involve 3 neurons - a **sensory neuron**, a **relay neuron** and a **motor neuron**. A stimulus, a pin in the paw for example, initiates an impulse in the sensory neuron that passes via a synapse to the relay neuron situated in the spinal cord and then via another synapse to the motor neurone. This transmits the impulse to the muscle causing it to contract and remove the paw from the pin.
- The nervous system is divided into 2 parts: the **central nervous system**, consisting of the brain and spinal cord and the **peripheral nervous system** consisting of nerves connected to the brain and spinal cord. The **autonomic nervous system** is considered to be part of the peripheral nervous system.
- The brain consists of three major regions: 1. the **fore brain** which includes the **cerebral hemispheres** (or **cerebrum**), **hypothalamus** and **pituitary gland**; 2. the **hindbrain** or **brain stem** containing the **medulla oblongata** and 3. the **cerebellum**.
- Protective membranes known as the **meninges** surround the brain and spinal cord.
- There are 12 pairs of cranial nerves that include the optic, olfactory, acoustic and **vagus** nerves.
- The **spinal cord** is a cable of nerve tissue surrounded by meninges passing from the brain to the end of the tail. **Spinal nerves** emerge by a **ventral** and **dorsal root** between each vertebra and connect the spinal cord with organs and muscles.
- The **autonomic nervous system** controls internal body functions not under conscious control. It is divided into 2 parts with 2 different functions: the **sympathetic nervous system** that is involved in the flight and fight response including increased heart rate, bronchial dilation, dilation of the pupil and decreased gut activity. The **parasympathetic nervous system** is associated with decreased heart rate, pupil constriction and increased gut activity.

Worksheet

Nervous System Worksheet [2]

Test Yourself

1. Add the following labels to this diagram of a motor neuron.

    cell body | nucleus | axon | dendrites | myelin sheath | muscle fibres

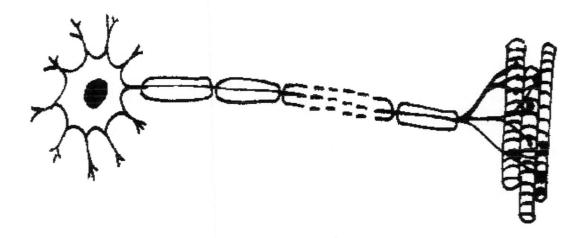

2. What is a synapse?

3. What is a reflex?

4. Rearrange the parts of a reflex arc given below in the order in which the nerve impulse travels from the sense organ to the muscle.

    sense organ | relay neuron | motor neuron | sensory neuron | muscle fibres

5. Add the following labels to the diagram of the dog's brain shown below.

    cerebellum | cerebral hemisphere | cerebral cortex | pituitary gland | medulla oblongata

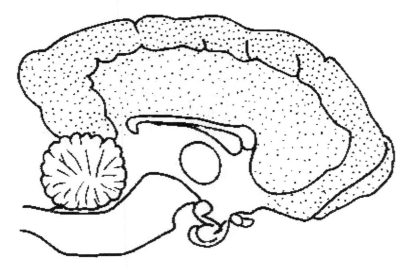

6. What is the function of the meninges that cover the brain and spinal cord

7. Give 3 effects of the action of the sympathetic nervous system.

Test Yourself Answers

Websites

- http://en.wikipedia.org/wiki/Neuron Wikipedia. Lots of good information here but as usual a warning that there are terms and concepts that are beyond the scope of this course. Also try 'reflex action' ; 'autonomic nervous system' ;

- http://images.google.co.nz/imgres?imgurl=http://static.howstuffworks.com/gif/brain-neuron.gif& imgrefurl=http://science.howstuffworks.com/brain1.htm&h=296&w=394&sz=17&hl=en&start=5& tbnid=LWLRI9lW_5PZhM:&tbnh=93&tbnw=124&prev=/ images%3Fq%3Dneuron%26svnum%3D10%26hl%3Den%26lr%3D%26sa%3DN How Stuff Works. This site is for the neuron but try 'neuron types', 'brain parts' and 'balancing act' too.

- http://www.bbc.co.uk/schools/gcsebitesize/flash/bireflexarc.swf Reflex Arc. Nice clear and simple animation of a reflex arc.

Glossary

- Link to Glossary [4]

References

[1] http://flickr.com/photos/royalty-free-images/139764662/
[2] http://www.wikieducator.org/Nervous_System_Worksheet

Anatomy and Physiology of Animals/Nervous System/Test Yourself Answers

1. Add the following labels to this diagram of a motor neuron.

cell body | nucleus | axon | dendrites | myelin sheath | muscle fibres

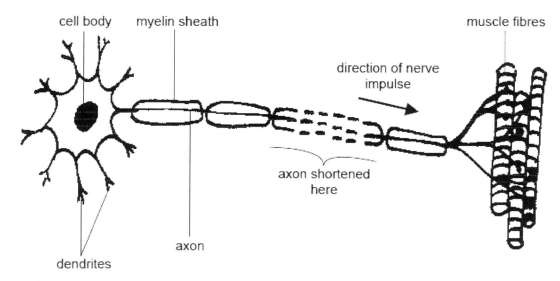

2. What is a synapse?

A synapse is where two adjacent neurons connect.

3. What is a reflex?

A reflex is an automatic response to a stimulus.

4. Rearrange the parts of a reflex arc given below in the order in which the nerve impulse travels from the sense organ to the muscle.

sense organ | relay neuron | motor neuron | sensory neuron | muscle fibres

The nerve impulse travels from the sense organ to the sensory neuron to the relay neuron to the motor neuron to the muscle fibres.

5. Add the following labels to the diagram of the dog's brain shown below.

cerebellum | cerebral hemisphere | cerebral cortex | pituitary gland | medulla oblongata

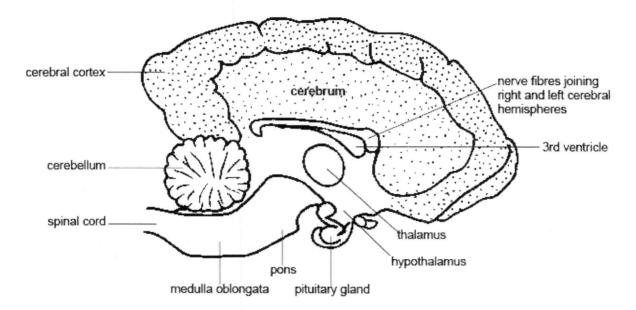

6. What is the function of the meninges that cover the brain and spinal cord

The meninges protect the brain and spinal cord.

7. Give 3 effects of the action of the sympathetic nervous system.

The sympathetic nervous system increases the heart rate, the rate of breathing, the blood flow to skeletal muscles and causes the pupils of the eye to dilate.

Anatomy and Physiology of Animals/The Senses

Objectives

After completing this section, you should know:

- that the general senses of touch, pressure, pain etc. are situated in the dermis of the skin and in the body
- that the special senses include those of smell, taste, sight, hearing, and balance
- the main structures of the eye and their functions
- the route taken by light through the eye to the retina
- the role of the rods and cones in the retina
- the advantages of binocular vision
- the main structures of the ear and their functions
- the route taken by sound waves through the ear to the cochlea
- the role of the vestibular organ (semicircular canals and otolith organ) in maintaining balance and posture

The Sense Organs

Sense organs allow animals to sense changes in the environment around them and in their bodies so that they can respond appropriately. They enable animals to avoid hostile environments, sense the presence of predators and find food.

Chapter 15 | The Senses

original image by miss pupik [1] cc by

Animals can sense a wide range of stimuli that includes, touch, pressure, pain, temperature, chemicals, light, sound, movement and position of the body. Some animals can sense electric and magnetic fields. All sense organs respond to stimuli by producing nerve impulses that travel to the brain via a sensory nerve. The impulses are then processed and interpreted in the brain as pain, sight, sound, taste etc.

The senses are often divided into two groups:

1. The **general senses** of touch, pressure, pain and temperature that are distributed fairly evenly through the skin. Some are found in muscles and within joints.

2. The **special senses** which include the senses of smell, taste, sight, hearing and balance. The special sense organs may be quite complex in structure.

Touch And Pressure

Within the dermis of the skin are numerous modified nerve endings that are sensitive to touch and pressure. The roots of hairs may also be well supplied with sensory receptors that inform the animal that it is in contact with an object (see diagram 15.1). Whiskers are specially modified hairs.

Pain

Receptors that sense pain are found in almost every tissue of the body. They tell the animal that tissues are dangerously hot, cold, compressed or stretched or that there is not enough blood flowing in them. The animal may then be able to respond and protect itself from further damage

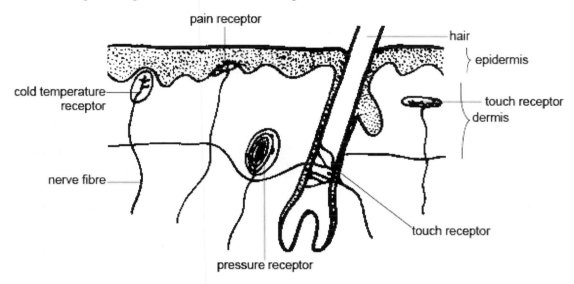

Diagram 15.1 - The general senses in the skin

Temperature

Nerve endings in the skin respond to hot and cold stimuli (See diagram 15.1).

Awareness Of Limb Position

There are sense organs in the muscles, tendons and joints that send continuous impulses to the brain that tell it where each limb is. This information allows the animal to place its limbs accurately and know their exact position without having to watch them.

Smell

Animals use the sense of smell to locate food, mark territory, identify their own offspring and the presence and sexual condition of a potential mate. The organ of smell (**olfactory organ**) is located in the nose and responds to chemicals in the air. It consists of modified nerve cells that have several tiny hairs on the surface. These emerge from the epithelium on the roof of the nose cavity into the mucus that lines it. As the animal breathes, chemicals in the air dissolve in the mucus. When the sense cell responds to a particular molecule, it fires an impulse that travels along the **olfactory nerve** to the brain where it is interpreted as an odour (see diagram 15.2).

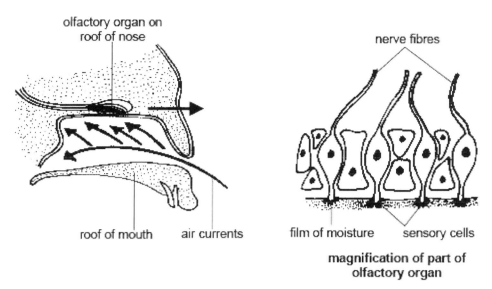

Diagram 15.2 - The olfactory organ - the sense of smell

The olfactory sense in humans is rudimentary compared to that of many animals. Carnivores that hunt have a very highly developed sensitivity to scents. For example a polar bear can smell out a dead seal 20 km away and a bloodhound can distinguish between the trails of different people although it may sometimes be confused by the criss-crossing trail of identical twins.

Snakes and lizards detect odours by means of **Jacobson's organ**. This is situated on the roof of the mouth and consists of pits containing sensory cells. When snakes flick out their forked tongues they are smelling the air by carrying the molecules in it to the Jacobson's organ.

Taste

The sense of taste allows animals to detect and identify dissolved chemicals. In reptiles, birds, and mammals the taste receptors (**taste buds**) are found mainly to the upper surface of the tongue. They consist of pits containing sensory cells arranged rather like the segments of an orange (see diagram 15.3). Each receptor cell has a tiny "hair" that projects into the saliva to sense the chemicals dissolved in it.

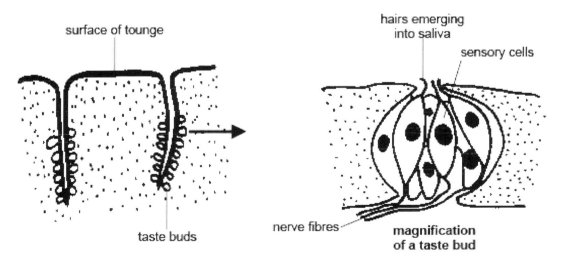

Diagram 15.3. Taste buds on the tongue

The sense of taste is quite restricted. Humans can only distinguish four different tastes (sweet, sour, bitter and salt) and what we normally think of as taste is mainly the sense of smell. Food is quite tasteless when the nose is blocked and cats often refuse to eat when this happens.

Sight

The eyes are the organs of sight. They consist of spherical **eyeballs** situated in deep depressions in the skull called the **orbits**. They are attached to the wall of the orbit by six muscles, which move the eyeball. Upper and lower **eyelids** cover the eyes during sleep and protect them from foreign objects or too much light, and spread the tears over their surface.

The **nictitating membrane** or **haw** is a transparent sheet that moves sideways across the eye from the inner corner, cleansing and moistening the cornea without shutting out the light. It is found in birds, crocodiles, frogs and fish as well as marsupials like the kangaroo. It is rare in mammals but can be seen in cats and dogs by gently opening the eye when it is asleep. **Eyelashes** also protect the eyes from the sun and foreign objects.

Structure of the Eye

Lining the eyelids and covering the front of the eyeball is a thin epithelium called the **conjunctiva**. Conjunctivitis is inflammation of this membrane. **Tear glands** that open just under the top eyelid secrete a salty solution that keeps the exposed part of the eye moist, washes away dust and contains an enzyme that destroys bacteria.

The wall of the eyeball is composed of three layers (see diagram 15.4). From the outside these are the **sclera**, the **choroid** and the **retina**.

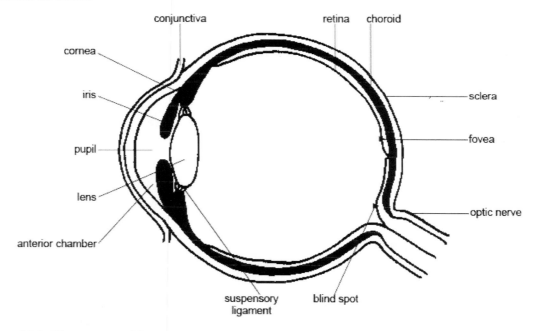

Diagram 15.4 - The structure of the eye

The **sclera** is a tough fibrous layer that protects the eyeball and gives it rigidity. At the front of the eye the sclera is visible as the "**white**" of the eye, which is modified as the transparent **cornea** through which the light rays have to pass to enter the eye. The cornea helps focus light that enters the eye.

The **choroid** lies beneath the sclera. It contains a network of blood vessels that supply the eye with oxygen and nutrients. Its inner surface is highly pigmented and absorbs stray light rays. In nocturnal animals like the cat and possum this highly pigmented layer reflects light as a means of conserving light. This is what makes them shine when caught in car headlights.

At the front of the eye the choroid becomes the **iris**. This is the coloured part of the eye that controls the amount of light entering the **pupil** of the eye. In dim light the pupil is wide open so as much light as possible enters while in bright light the pupils contract to protect the retina from damage by excess light.

The **pupil** in most animals is circular but in many nocturnal animals it is a slit that can close completely. This helps protect the extra-sensitive light sensing tissues of animals like the cat and possum from bright sunlight.

The inner layer lining the inside of the eye is the **retina**. This contains the light sensing cells called **rods** and **cones** (see diagram 15.5).

The **rod cells** are long and fat and are sensitive to dim light but cannot detect colour. They contain large amounts of a pigment that changes when exposed to light. This pigment comes from vitamin A found in carrots etc. A deficiency of this vitamin causes night blindness. So your mother was right when she told you to eat your carrots as they would help you see in the dark!

The **cone cells** provide colour vision and allow animals to see details. Most are found in the centre of the retina and they are most densely concentrated in a small area called the **fovea**. This is the area of sharpest vision, where the words you are reading at this moment are focussed on your retina.

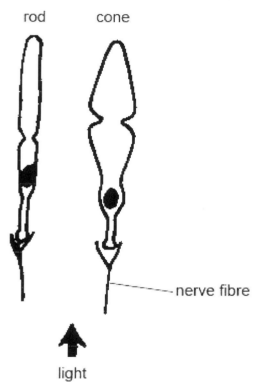

Diagram 15.5 - A rod and cone from the retina

The nerve fibres from the cells of the retina join and leave the eye via the **optic nerve**. There are no rods or cones here and it is a **blind spot**. The optic nerve passes through the back of the orbit and enters the brain.

The **lens** is situated just behind the pupil and the iris. It is a crystalline structure with no blood vessels and is held in position by a ligament. This is attached to a muscle, which changes the shape of the lens so both near and distant objects can be focussed by the eye. This ability to change the focus of the lens is called **accommodation**. In many mammals the muscles that bring about accommodation are poorly developed, Rats, cows and dogs, for example, are thought to be unable to focus clearly on near objects.

In old age and certain diseases the lens may become cloudy resulting in blurred vision. This is called a **cataract**. Within the eyeball are two cavities, the **anterior and posterior chambers**, separated by the lens. They contain fluids the **aqueous and vitreous humours**respectively, that maintain the shape of the eyeball and help press the retina firmly against the choroid so clear images are seen.

How The Eye Sees

Eyes work quite like a camera. Light rays from an object enter the eye and are focused on the retina (the "film") at the back of the eye. The cornea, the lens and the fluid within the eye all help to focus the light. They do this by bending the light rays so that light from the object falls on the retina. This bending of light is called **refraction**. The light stimulates the light sensitive cells of the retina and nerve impulses are produced that pass down the optic nerve to the brain (see diagram 15.6).

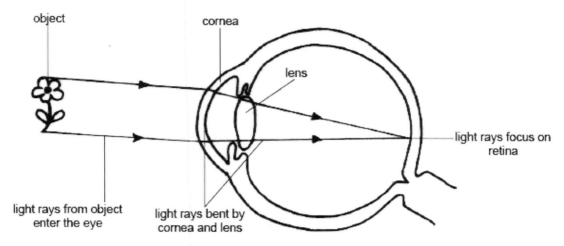

Diagram 15.6 - How the light travels from the object to the retina of the eye

Colour Vision In Animals

As mentioned before, the retina has two different kinds of cells that are stimulated by light - *'rods'* and *'cones'*. In humans and higher primates like baboons and gorillas the rods function in dim light and do not perceive colour, while the cones are stimulated by bright light and perceive details and colour.

Other mammals have very few cones in their retinas and it is believed that they see no or only a limited range of colour. It is, of course, difficult to find out exactly what animals do see. It is thought that deer, rats, and rabbits and nocturnal animals like the cat are colour-blind, and dogs probably see green and blue. Some fish and most birds seem to have better colour vision than humans and they use colour, often very vivid ones, for recognizing each other as well as for courtship and protection.

Binocular Vision

Animals like cats that hunt have eyes placed on the front of the head in such a way that both eyes see the same wide area but from slightly different angles (see diagram 15.7). This is called binocular vision. **Its main advantage is that it enables the animals to estimate the distance to the prey so they can chase it and pounce accurately.**

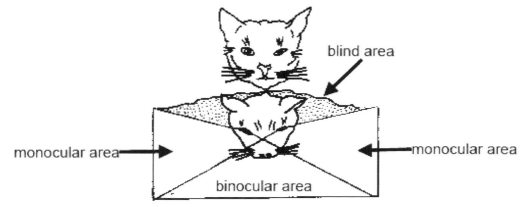

Diagram 15.7 - Well developed binocular vision in predator animals like the cat

In contrast plant-eating prey animals like the rabbit and deer need to have a wide panoramic view so they can see predators approaching. They therefore have eyes placed on the side of the head, each with its own field of vision (see diagram 15.8). They have only a very small area of binocular vision in front of the head but are extremely sensitive to movement.

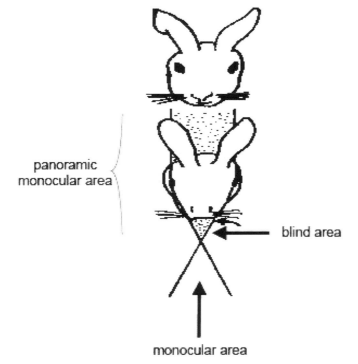

Diagram 15.8 - Panoramic monocular vision in prey animals like the rabbit

Hearing

Animals use the sense of hearing for many different purposes. It is used to sense danger and enemies, to detect prey, to identify prospective mates and to communicate within social groups. Some animals (e.g. most bats and dolphins) use sound to "see" by echolocation. By sending out a cry and interpreting the echo, they sense obstacles or potential prey.

Structure of the Ear

Most of the ear, the organ of hearing, is hidden from view within the boney skull. It consists of three main regions: the **outer ear, the middle ear** and the **inner ear** (see diagram 15.9).

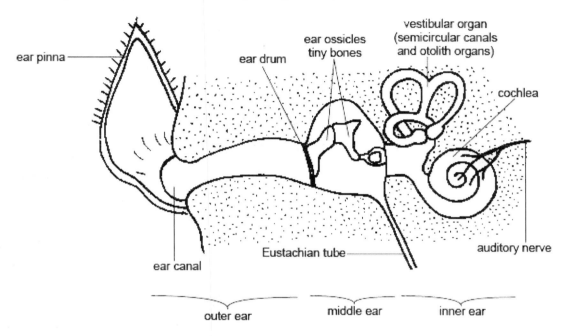

Diagram 15.9 - The ear

The **outer ear** consists of an **ear canal** leading inwards to a thin membrane known as the **eardrum**or **tympanic membrane** that stretches across the canal. Many animals have an external ear flap or **pinna** to collect and funnel the sound into the ear canal. The pinnae (plural of pinna) usually face forwards on the head but many animals can swivel them towards the source of the sound.

In dogs the ear canal is long and bent and often traps wax or provides an ideal habitat for mites, yeast and bacteria.

The **middle ear** consists of a cavity in the skull that is connected to the **pharynx** (throat) by a long narrow tube called the **Eustachian tube**. This links the middle ear to the outside air so that the air pressure on both sides of the eardrum can be kept the same. Everyone knows the uncomfortable feeling (and affected hearing) that occurs when you drive down a steep hill and the unequal air pressures on the two sides of the eardrum cause it to distort. The discomfort is relieved when you swallow because the Eustachian tubes open and the pressure on either side equalises.

Within the cavity of the middle ear are three of the smallest bones in the body, the **auditory ossicles**. They are known as the hammer, the anvil and the stirrup because of their resemblance to the shape of these objects. These tiny bones articulate (move against) each other and transfer the vibrations of the eardrum to the membrane covering the opening to the inner ear.

The **inner ear** is a complicated series of fluid-filled tubes imbedded in the bone of the skull. It consists of two main parts. These are the **cochlea** where sound waves are converted to nerve impulses and the **vestibular organ** that is associated with the sense of balance and has no role in hearing (see later).

The **cochlea** looks rather like a coiled up snail shell. Within it there are specialised cells with fine hairs on their surface that respond to the movement of the fluid within the cochlea by producing nervous impulses that travel to the brain along the **auditory nerve**.

How The Ear Hears

Sound waves can be thought of as vibrations in the air. They are collected by the ear pinna and pass down the ear canal where they cause the eardrum to vibrate. (An interesting fact is that when you are listening to someone speaking your eardrum vibrates at exactly the same rate as the vocal cords of the person speaking to you).

The vibration of the eardrum sets the three tiny bones in the middle ear moving against each other so that the vibration is transferred to the membrane covering the opening to the inner ear. As well as transferring the vibration, the tiny ear bones also amplify it. The three tiny bones are called the stirrup, anvil, and hammer. They were called such of their form. In the human ear this amplification is about 20 times while in desert-dwelling animals like the kangaroo rat it is 100 times. This acute hearing warns them of the approach of predators like owls and snakes, even in the dark.

The vibration causes waves in the fluid in the inner ear that pass down the cochlea. These waves stimulate the tiny hair cells to produce nerve impulses that travel via the auditory nerve to the cerebral cortex of the brain where they are interpreted as sound.

To summarise: The route sound waves take as they pass through the ear is: **External ear | tympanic membrane | ear ossicles | inner ear |cochlear | hair cells**

The hair cells generate a nerve impulse that travels down the auditory nerve to the brain.

Remember that sound waves do not pass along the Eustachian tube. Its function is to equalise the air pressure on either side of the tympanic membrane.

Balance

The **vestibular organ** of the inner ear helps an animal maintain its posture and keep balanced by monitoring the movement and position of the head. It consists of two structures - the **semicircular canals** and the **otolith organs**.

The **semicircular canals** (see diagram 15.10) respond to movement of the body. They tell an animal whether it is moving up or down, left or right. They consist of three canals set in three different planes at right angles to each other so that movement in any direction can be registered. The canals contain fluid and sense cells with fine hairs that project into the fluid. When the head moves the fluid swirls in the canals and stimulates the hair cells. These send nerve impulses along the **vestibular nerve** to the **cerebellum**.

Note that the semicircular canals register acceleration and deceleration as well as changes in direction but do not respond to movement that is at a constant speed.

The **otolith organs** are sometimes known as gravity receptors. They tell you if your head is tilted or if you are standing on your head. They consist of bulges at the base of the semi circular canals that contain hair cells that are covered by a mass of jelly containing tiny pieces of chalk called **otoliths** (see diagram 15.10). When the head is tilted, or moved suddenly, the otoliths pull on the hair cells, which produce a nerve impulse. This travels down the **vestibular nerve** to the **cerebellum**. By coordinating the nerve impulses from the semicircular canals and otolith organs the cerebellum helps the animal keep its balance.

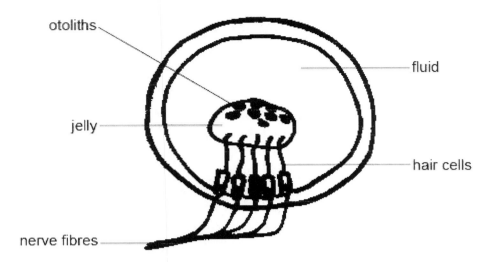

otoliths

fluid

jelly

hair cells

nerve fibres

Diagram 15.10 - Otolith Organs

Summary

- Receptors for touch, pressure, pain and temperature are found in the skin. Receptors in the muscles, tendons and joints inform the brain of limb position.
- The **olfactory organ** in the nose responds to chemicals in the air i.e. smell.
- **Taste buds** on the tongue respond to a limited range of chemicals dissolved in saliva.
- The eyes are the organs of sight. Spherical **eyeballs** situated in orbits in the skull have walls composed of 3 layers.
- The tough outer **sclera** protects and holds the shape of the eyeball. At the front it becomes visible as the white of the eye and the transparent **cornea** that allows light to enter the eye.
- The middle layer is the **choroid**. It most animals it absorbs stray light rays but in nocturnal animal it is reflective to conserve light. At the front of the eye it becomes the **iris** with muscles to control the size of the **pupil** and hence the amount of light entering the eye.
- The inner layer is the **retina** containing the light receptor cells: the **rods** for black and white vision in dim light and the **cones** for colour and detailed vision. Nerve impulses generated by these cells leave the eye for the brain via the **optic nerve**.
- The **lens** (with the cornea) helps focus the light rays on the retina. Muscles alter the shape of the lens to allow near and far objects to be focussed.
- **Aqueous humour** fills the space immediately behind the cornea and keeps it in shape and **vitreous humour**, a transparent jelly-like substance, fills the space behind the lens allowing light rays to pass through to the retina.
- The ear is the organ of hearing and balance.
- The external **pinna** helps funnel sound waves into the ear and locate the direction of the sound. The sound waves travel down the external **ear canal** to the **eardrum** or **tympanic membrane** causing it to vibrate. This vibration is transferred to the **auditory ossicles** of the middle ear which themselves transfer it to the inner ear. Here receptors in the **cochlea** respond by generating nerve impulses that travel to the brain via the **auditory** (acoustic) nerve.
- The **Eustachian tube** connects the middle ear with the pharynx to equalise air pressure on either side of the tympanic membrane.
- The **vestibular organ** of the inner ear is concerned with maintaining balance and posture. It consists of the **semicircular canals** and the **otolith organs**.

Worksheet

Senses Worksheet [2]

Test Yourself

1. Where are the organs that sense pain, pressure and temperature found?

2. Which sense organ responds to chemicals in the air?

3. Match the words in the list below with the following descriptions.

optic nerve | choroid | cornea | aqueous humor | retina | cones | iris | vitreous humour | sclera | lens

a) Focuses light rays on the retina.

b) Respond to colour and detail.

c) Outer coat of the eyeball.

d) Carries nerve impulses from the retina to the brain.

e) The chamber behind the lens is filled with this.

f) This layer of the eyeball reflects light in nocturnal animals like the cat.

g) This is the transparent window at the front of the eye.

h) This constricts in bright light to reduce the amount of light entering the eye.

i) The light rays are focused on here by the lens and cornea.

j) The chamber in front of the lens is filled with this.

4. Add the following labels to the diagram of the ear below.

pinna | Eustachian tube | cochlea | tympanic membrane | external ear canal | ear ossicles | semicircular canals

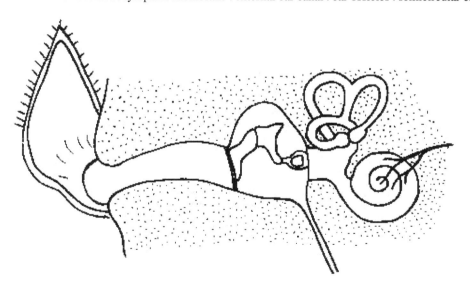

5. What is the role of the Eustachian tube?

6. What do the ear ossicles do?

7. What is the role of the semicircular canals?

Senses Test Yourself Answers

Websites

- http://en.wikipedia.org/wiki/Sense Wikipedia. The old faithful. You can explore here to your hearts desire. Try 'eye', 'ear', 'taste' etc. but also 'equilibrioception', and 'echolocation'.

- http://www.bbc.co.uk/science/humanbody/body/factfiles/smell/smell_ani_f5.swf BBC Science and Nature. BBC animation of (human) olfactory organ and smelling.

- http://www.bbc.co.uk/science/humanbody/body/factfiles/taste/taste_ani_f5.swf BBC Science. BBC animation of (human) taste buds and tasting.

- http://www.bishopstopford.com/faculties/science/arthur/Eye%20Drag%20%26%20Drop.swf Eye Diagram. A diagram of the eye to label and test your knowledge.

- http://www.bbc.co.uk/science/humanbody/body/factfiles/hearing/hearing_animation.shtml BBC on Hearing. BBC animation of hearing. Well worth looking at.

- http://www.wisc-online.com/objects/index_tj.asp?objid=AP1502 Ear Animation. Another great animation of the ear and hearing.

- http://www.bbc.co.uk/science/humanbody/body/factfiles/balance/balance_ani_f5.swf BBC Balance Animation. An animation of the action of the otolith organ (called macula in this animation)

Glossary

- Link to Glossary [4]

References

[1] http://flickr.com/photos/miss_pupik/5350317/

[2] http://www.wikieducator.org/Special_Senses_Worksheet

Anatomy and Physiology of Animals/The Senses/Senses Test Yourself Answers

1. Where are the organs that sense pain, pressure and temperature found?

   The organs that sense pain, pressure and temperature are found in the dermis of the skin.

2. Which sense organ responds to chemicals in the air?

   The olfactory organ in the nose responds to chemicals in the air.

3. Match the words in the list below with the following descriptions.

   optic nerve | choroid | cornea | aqueous humor | retina | cones | iris | vitreous humour | sclera | lens

   a) Focuses light rays on the retina - *Lens*

   b) Respond to colour and detail - *Cones*

   c) Outer coat of the eyeball - *Sclera*

   d) Carries nerve impulses from the retina to the brain - *Optic nerve*

   e) The chamber behind the lens is filled with this - *Vitreous humour*

   f) This layer of the eyeball reflects light in nocturnal animals like the cat - *Choroid*

   g) This is the transparent window at the front of the eye. *Cornea*

   h) This constricts in bright light to reduce the amount of light entering the eye - *Iris*

   i) The light rays are focused on here by the lens and cornea - *Retina*

   j) The chamber in front of the lens is filled with this - *Aqueous humour*

4. Add the following labels to the diagram of the ear below.

   pinna | Eustachian tube | cochlea | tympanic membrane | external ear canal | ear ossicles | semicircular canals

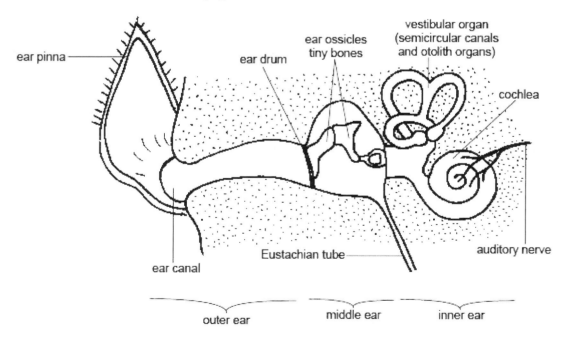

5. What is the role of the Eustachian tube?

   The Eustachian tube equalises air pressure on either side of the tympanic membrane.

6. What do the ear ossicles do?

The ear ossicles transmit vibrations across the middle ear to the inner ear.

7. What is the role of the semicircular canals?

The semicircular canals respond to movement of the head including acceleration and slowing down.

Anatomy and Physiology of Animals/Endocrine System

Objectives

After completing this section, you should know:

- The characteristics of endocrine glands and hormones
- The position of the main endocrine glands in the body
- The relationship between the pituitary gland and the hypothalamus
- The main hormones produced by the two parts of the pituitary gland and their effects on the body
- The main hormones produced by the pineal, thyroid, parathyroid and adrenal glands, the pancreas, ovary and testis and their effects on the body
- What is meant by homeostasis and feedback control
- The homeostatic mechanisms that allow an animal to control its body temperature, water balance, blood volume and acid/base balance

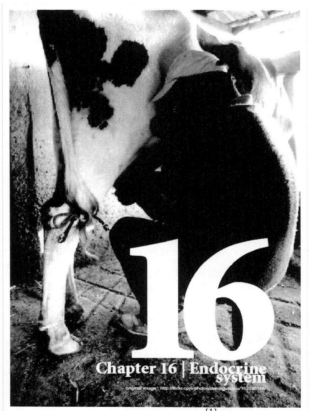

original image by Denis Gustavo [1] cc by

The Endocrine System

In order to survive, animals must constantly adapt to changes in the environment. The **nervous** and **endocrine systems** both work together to bring about this adaptation. In general the nervous system responds rapidly to short-term changes by sending electrical impulses along nerves and the endocrine system brings about longer-term adaptations by sending out chemical messengers called hormones into the blood stream.

For example, think about what happens when a male and female cat meet under your bedroom window at night. The initial response of both cats may include spitting, fighting and spine tingling yowling - all brought about by the nervous system. Fear and stress then activates the adrenal glands to secrete the hormone **adrenaline** which increases the heart and respiratory rates. If mating occurs, other hormones stimulate the release of ova from the ovary of the female and a range of different hormones maintains pregnancy, delivery of the kittens and lactation.

Endocrine Glands And Hormones

Hormones are chemicals that are secreted by **endocrine glands**. Unlike exocrine glands (see chapter 5), endocrine glands have no ducts, but release their secretions directly into the blood system, which carries them throughout the body. However, hormones only affect the specific **target organs** that recognize them. For example, although it is carried to virtually every cell in the body, **follicle stimulating hormone** (FSH), released from the **anterior pituitary gland**, only acts on the follicle cells of the ovaries causing them to develop.

A nerve impulse travels rapidly and produces an almost instantaneous response but one that lasts only briefly. In contrast, hormones act more slowly and their effects may be long lasting. Target cells respond to minute quantities of hormones and the concentration in the blood is always extremely low. However, target cells are sensitive to subtle changes in hormone concentration and the endocrine system regulates processes by changing the rate of hormone secretion.

The main endocrine glands in the body are the **pituitary, pineal, thyroid, parathyroid**, and **adrenal glands**, the **pancreas, ovaries** and **testes**. Their positions in the body are shown in diagram 16.1.

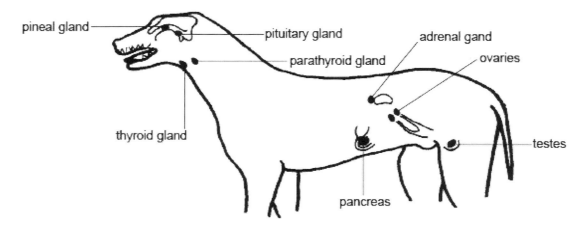

Diagram 16.1 - The main endocrine organs of the body

The Pituitary Gland And Hypothalamus

The **pituitary gland** is a pea-sized structure that is attached by a stalk to the underside of the cerebrum of the brain (see diagram 16.2). It is often called the "master" endocrine gland because it controls many of the other endocrine glands in the body. However, we now know that the pituitary gland is itself controlled by the **hypothalamus**. This small but vital region of the brain lies just above the pituitary and provides the link between the nervous and endocrine systems. It controls the **autonomic nervous system**, produces a range of hormones and regulates the secretion of many others from the pituitary gland (see Chapter 7 for more information on the hypothalamus).

The pituitary gland is divided into two parts with different functions - the **anterior** and **posterior pituitary** (see diagram 16.3).

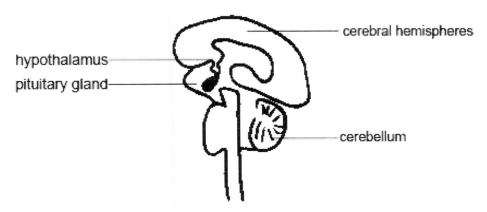

Diagram 16.2 - The position of the pituitary gland and hypothalamus

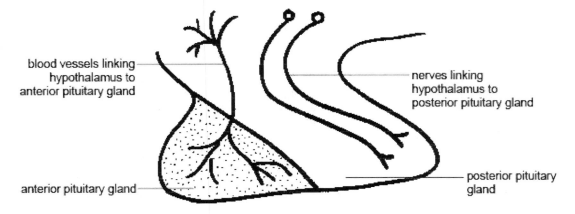

Diagram 16.3 - The anterior and posterior pituitary

The **anterior pituitary gland** secretes hormones that regulate a wide range of activities in the body. These include:

1. **Growth hormone** that stimulates body growth.

2. **Prolactin** that initiates milk production.

3. **Follicle stimulating hormone (FSH)** that stimulates the development of the **follicles** of the ovaries. These then secrete **oestrogen** (see chapter 6). In the

The Pineal Gland

The **pineal gland** is found deep within the brain (see diagram 16.4). It is sometimes known as the 'third eye" as it responds to light and day length. It produces the hormone **melatonin**, which influences the development of sexual maturity and the seasonality of breeding and hibernation.

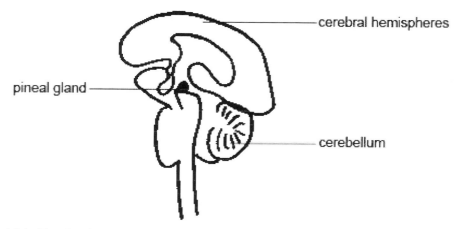

Diagram 16.4 - The pineal gland

The Thyroid Gland

The **thyroid gland** is situated in the neck, just in front of the windpipe or trachea (see diagram 16.5). It produces the hormone **thyroxine**, which influences the rate of growth and development of young animals. In mature animals it increases the rate of chemical reactions in the body.

Thyroxine consists of 60% **iodine** and too little in the diet can cause **goitre**, an enlargement of the thyroid gland. Many inland soils in New Zealand contain almost no iodine so goitre can be common in stock when iodine supplements are not given. To add to the problem, chemicals called **goitrogens** that occur naturally in plants like kale that belong to the **cabbage family**, can also cause goitre even when there is adequate iodine available.

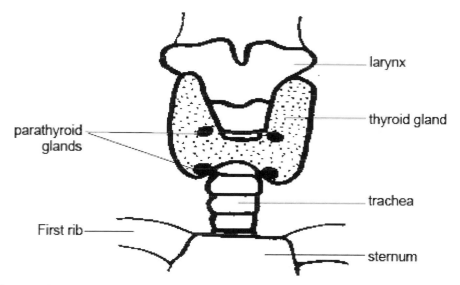

Diagram 16.5 - The thyroid and parathyroid glands

The Parathyroid Glands

The **parathyroid glands** are also found in the neck just behind the thyroid glands (see diagram 16.5). They produce the hormone **parathormone** that regulates the amount of **calcium** in the blood and influences the excretion of **phosphates** in the urine.

The Adrenal Gland

The **adrenal glands** are situated on the cranial surface of the kidneys (see diagram 16.6). There are two parts to this endocrine gland, an outer **cortex** and an inner **medulla**.

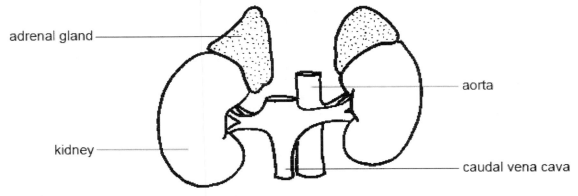

Diagram 16.6 - The adrenal glands

The **adrenal cortex** produces several hormones. These include:

1. **Aldosterone** that regulates the concentration of **sodium and potassium** in the blood by controlling the amounts that are secreted or reabsorbed in the kidney tubules.

2. **Cortisone** and **hydrocortisone** (cortisol) that have complex effects on glucose, protein and fat metabolism. In general they increase metabolism. They are also often administered to animals to counteract allergies and for treating arthritic and rheumatic conditions. However, prolonged use should be avoided if possible as they can increase weight and reduce the ability to heal.

3. **Male and female sex hormones** similar to those secreted by the ovaries and testes.

The hormones secreted by the adrenal cortex also play a part in "**general adaptation syndrome**" which occurs in situations of prolonged stress.

The **adrenal medulla** secretes **adrenalin** (also called **epinephrine**). Adrenalin is responsible for the so-called flight fight, fright response that prepares the animal for emergencies. Faced with a perilous situation the animal needs to either fight or make a rapid escape. To do either requires instant energy, particularly in the skeletal muscles. Adrenaline increases the amount of blood reaching them by causing their blood vessels to dilate and the heart to beat faster. An increased rate of breathing increases the amount of oxygen in the blood and glucose is released from the liver to provide the fuel for energy production. Sweating increases to keep the muscles cool and the pupils of the eye dilate so the animal has a wide field of view. Functions like digestion and urine production that are not critical to immediate survival slow down as blood vessels to these parts constrict.

Note that the effects of adrenalin are similar to those of the sympathetic nervous system.

The Pancreas

In most animals the **pancreas** is an oblong, pinkish organ that lies in the first bend of the small intestine (see diagram 16.7). In rodents and rabbits, however, it is spread thinly through the mesentery and is sometimes difficult to see.

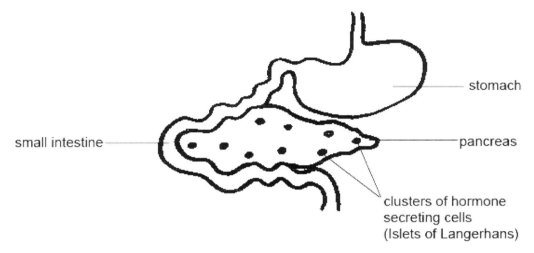

Diagram 16.7 - The pancreas

Most of the pancreas acts as an **exocrine gland** producing digestive enzymes that are secreted into the small intestine. The endocrine part of the organ consists of small clusters of cells (called **Islets of Langerhans**) that secrete the hormone **insulin**. This hormone regulates the amount of **glucose** in the blood by increasing the rate at which glucose is converted to glycogen in the liver and the movement of glucose from the blood into cells.

In **diabetes mellitus** the pancreas produces insufficient insulin and glucose levels in the blood can increase to a dangerous level. A major symptom of this condition is glucose in the urine.

The Ovaries

The ovaries, located in the lower abdomen, produce two important sex hormones.

1. The **follicle cells**, under the influence of **FSH** (see the pituitary gland above), produce **oestrogen**, which stimulates the development of female sexual characteristics - the mammary glands, generally smaller build of female animals etc. It also stimulates the thickening of the lining of the uterus in preparation for pregnancy (see chapter 13).

2. **Progesterone** is produced by the **corpus luteum**, the endocrine gland that develops in the empty follicle following ovulation (see chapter 13). It promotes the further preparation of the uterine lining for pregnancy and prevents the uterus contracting until the baby is born.

The Testes

Cells around the sperm producing ducts of the testis produce the hormone **testosterone**. This stimulates the development of the male reproductive system and the male sexual characteristics - generally larger body of male animals, mane in lions, tusks in boars, etc.

Summary

- **Hormones** are chemicals that are released into the blood by **endocrine glands** i.e. Glands with no ducts. Hormones act on specific **target organs** that recognize them.
- The main endocrine glands in the body are the **hypothalamus, pituitary, pineal, thyroid, parathyroid** and **adrenal glands,** the **pancreas, ovaries** and **testes**.
- The **hypothalamus** is situated under the **cerebrum** of the brain. It produces or controls many of the hormones released by the pituitary gland lying adjacent to it.
- The **pituitary gland** is divided into two parts: the **anterior pituitary** and the **posterior pituitary**.
- The **anterior pituitary** produces:
  - **Growth hormone** that stimulates body growth
  - **Prolactin** that initiates milk production
  - **Follicle stimulating hormone (FSH)** that stimulates the development of **ova**
  - **Luteinising hormone (LH)** that stimulates the development of the **corpus luteum**
  - Plus several other hormones
- The **posterior pituitary** releases:
  - **Antidiuretic hormone** (ADH) that regulates **water loss** and raises **blood pressure**
  - **Oxytocin** that stimulates milk "let down".
- The **pineal gland** in the brain produces **melatonin** that influences **sexual development** and **breeding cycles**.
- The **thyroid gland** located in the neck, produces thyroxine, which influences the **rate of growth** and **development** of young animals. Thyroxine consists of 60% **iodine**. Lack of iodine leads to **goitre**.
- The **parathyroid glands** situated adjacent to the thyroid glands in the neck produce **parathormone** that regulates blood **calcium** levels and the excretion of **phosphates**.
- The **adrenal gland** located adjacent to the kidneys is divided into the outer **cortex** and the inner **medulla**.
- The **adrenal cortex** produces:
  - **Aldosterone** that regulates the blood concentration of **sodium and potassium**
  - **Cortisone** and **hydrocortisone** that affect **glucose, protein** and **fat** metabolism
  - Male and female **sex hormones**
- The **adrenal medulla** produces **adrenalin** responsible for the **flight, fright, fight** response that prepares animals for emergencies.
- The **pancreas** that lies in the first bend of the small intestine produces **insulin** that regulates blood **glucose** levels.
- The **ovaries** are located in the lower abdomen produce 2 important sex hormones:
  - The **follicle cells** of the developing ova produce **oestrogen**, which controls the development of the **mammary glands** and prepares the uterus for pregnancy.
  - The **corpus luteum** that develops in the empty **follicle** after ovulation produces **progesterone**. This hormone further prepares the **uterus** for pregnancy and maintains the pregnancy.
- The **testes** produce **testosterone** that stimulates the development of the **male reproductive system** and **sexual characteristics**.

Homeostasis and Feedback Control

Animals can only survive if the environment within their bodies and their cells is kept constant and independent of the changing conditions in the external environment. As mentioned in module 1.6, the process by which this stability is maintained is called homeostasis. The body achieves this stability by constantly monitoring the internal conditions and if they deviate from the norm initiating processes that bring them back to it. This mechanism is called feedback control. For example, to maintain a constant body temperature the hypothalamus monitors the blood temperature and initiates processes that increase or decrease heat production by the body and loss from the skin so the optimum temperature is always maintained. The processes involved in the control of body temperature, water balance, blood loss and acid/base balance are summarized below.

Summary of Homeostatic Mechanisms

1. Temperature control

The biochemical and physiological processes in the cell are sensitive to temperature. The optimum body temperature is about 37⁰ C [99⁰ F] for mammals, and about 40⁰ C [104⁰ F] for birds. Biochemical processes in the cells, particularly in muscles and the liver, produce heat. The heat is distributed through the body by the blood and is lost mainly through the skin surface. The production of this heat and its loss through the skin is controlled by the hypothalamus in the brain which acts rather like a thermostat on an electric heater. .

(a) When the body temperature rises above the optimum, a decrease in temperature is achieved by:

* Sweating and panting to increase heat loss by evaporation.

* Expansion of the blood vessels near the skin surface so heat is lost to the air.

* Reducing muscle exertion to the minimum.

(b) When the body temperature falls below the optimum, an increase

* Moving to a heat source e.g. in the sun, out of the wind.

* Increasing muscular activity

* Shivering

* Making the hair stand on end by contraction of the hair erector muscles or fluffing of the feathers so there is an insulating layer of air around the body

* Constricting the blood vessels near the skin surface so heat loss to the air is decreased

2. Water balance

The concentration of the body fluids remains relatively constant irrespective of the diet or the quantity of water taken into the body by the animal. Water is lost from the body by many routes (see module 1.6) but the kidney is the main organ that influences the quantity that is lost. Again it is the hypothalamus that monitors the concentration of the blood and initiates the release of hormones from the posterior pituitary gland. These act on the kidney tubules to influence the amount of water (and sodium ions) absorbed from the fluid flowing along them.

(a) When the body fluids become too concentrated and the osmotic pressure too high, water retention in the kidney tubules can be achieved by:

* An increased production of antidiuretic hormone (ADH) from the posterior pituitary gland, which causes more water to be reabsorbed from the kidney tubules.

* A decreased blood pressure in the glomerulus of the kidney results in less fluid filtering through into the kidney tubules so less urine is produced.

(b) When the body fluids become too dilute and the osmotic pressure too low, water loss in the urine can be achieved by:

- A decrease in the secretion of ADH, so less water is reabsorbed from the kidney tubules and more concentrated urine is produced.
- An increase in the blood pressure in the glomerulus so more fluid filters into the kidney tubule and more urine is produced.
- An increase in sweating or panting that also increases the amount of water lost.

Another hormone, aldosterone, secreted by the cortex of the adrenal gland, also affects water balance indirectly. It does this by increasing the absorption of sodium ions (Na-) from the kidney tubules. This increases water retention since it increases the osmotic pressure of the fluids around the tubules and water therefore flows out of them by osmosis.

3. Maintenance of blood volume after moderate blood loss

Loss of blood or body fluids leads to decreased blood volume and hence decreased blood pressure. The result is that the blood system fails to deliver enough oxygen and nutrients to the cells, which stop functioning properly and may die. Cells of the brain are particularly vulnerable. This condition is known as shock.

If blood loss is not extreme, various mechanisms come into play to compensate and ensure permanent tissue damage does not occur. These mechanisms include:

- Increased thirst and drinking increases blood volume.
- Blood vessels in the skin and kidneys constrict to reduce the total volume of the blood system and hence retain blood pressure.
- Heart rate increases. This also increases blood pressure.
- Antidiuretic hormone (ADH) is released by the posterior pituitary gland. This increases water re-absorption in the collecting ducts of the kidney tubules so concentrated urine is produced and water loss is reduced. This helps maintain blood volume.
- Loss of fluid causes an increase in osmotic pressure of the blood. Proteins, mainly albumin, released into the blood by the liver further increase the osmotic pressure causing fluid from the tissues to be drawn into the blood by osmosis. This increases blood volume.
- Aldosterone, secreted by the adrenal cortex, increases the absorption of sodium ions (Na-) and water from the kidney tubules. This increases urine concentration and helps retain blood volume.

If blood or fluid loss is extreme and the blood volume falls by more than 15-25%, the above mechanisms are unable to compensate and the condition of the animal progressively deteriorates. The animal will die unless a vet administers fluid or blood.

4. Acid/ base balance

Biochemical reactions within the body are very sensitive to even small changes in acidity or alkalinity (i.e. pH) and any departure from the narrow limits disrupts the functioning of the cells. It is therefore important that the blood contains balanced quantities of acids and bases.

The normal pH of blood is in the range 7.35 to 7.45 and there are a number of mechanisms that operate to maintain the pH in this range. Breathing is one of these mechanisms.

Much of the carbon dioxide produced by respiration in cells is carried in the blood as carbonic acid. As the amount of carbon dioxide in the blood increases the blood becomes more acidic and the pH decreases. This is called acidosis and when severe can cause coma and death. On the other hand, alkalosis (blood that is too alkaline) causes over stimulation of the nervous system and when severe can lead to convulsions and death.

(a) When vigorous activity generating large quantities of carbon dioxide causes the blood to becomes too acidic it can be counteracted in two ways:

• By the rapid removal of carbon dioxide from the blood by deep, panting breaths

By the secretion of hydrogen ions (H+) into the urine by the kidney tubules.

(b) When over breathing or hyperventilation results in low levels of carbon dioxide in the blood and the blood is too alkaline, various mechanisms come into play to bring the pH back to within the normal range. These include:

• A slower rate of breathing

• A reduction in the amount of hydrogen ions (H+) secreted into the urine.

SUMMARY

Homeostasis is the maintenance of constant conditions within a cell or animal's body despite changes in the external environment.

Thebody temperature of mammals and birds is maintained at an optimum level by a variety of heat regulation mechanisms. These include:

• Seeking out warm areas,

• Adjusting activity levels,

blood vessesl on the body surface,

• Contraction of the erector muscles so hairs and feathers stand up to form an insulating layer,

• Shivering,

• Sweating and panting in dogs.

Animals maintain water balance by:

• adjusting level of antidiuretic hormone(ADH)

• adjusting level of aldosterone,

• adjusting blood flow to the kidneys

• adjusting the amount of water lost through sweating or panting.

Animals maintain blood volume after moderate blood loss by:

• Drinking,

• Constriction of blood vessels in the skin and kidneys,

• increasing heart rate,

• secretion of antidiuretic hormone

• secretion of aldosterone

• drawing fluid from the tissues into the blood by increasing the osmotic pressure of the blood.

Animals maintain the acid/base balance or pH of the blood by:

• Adjusting the rate of breathing and hence the amount of CO_2 removed from the blood.

• Adjusting the secretion of hydrogen ionsinto the urine.

Worksheet

Endocrine System Worksheet [2]

Test Yourself

1. What is Homeostasis?

2. Give 2 examples of homeostasis

3. List 3 ways in which animals keep their body temperature constant when the weather is hot

4. How does the kidney compensate when an animal is deprived of water to drink

5. After moderate blood loss, several mechanisms come into play to increase blood pressure and make up blood volume. 3 of these mechanisms are:

6. Describe how panting helps to reduce the acidity of the blood

Test Yourself Answers

Websites

• http://www.zerobio.com/drag_oa/endo.htm A drag and drop hormone and endocrine organ matching exercise.

• http://en.wikipedia.org/wiki/Endocrine_system Wikipedia. Much, much more than you ever need to know about hormones and the endocrine system but with a bit of discipline you can glean lots of useful information from this site.

Glossary

• Link to Glossary [4]

References

[1] http://flickr.com/photos/denisgustavo/183295115/
[2] http://www.wikieducator.org/Endocrine_System_Worksheet

Anatomy and Physiology of Animals/Endocrine System/Test Yourself Answers

1. What is Homeostasis?

Homeostasis is maintaining stability/constant conditions despite changes in the environment.

2. Give 2 examples of homeostasis.

Examples of homeostasis in an animal's body are the maintenance of a constant internal temperature despite fluctuations in the air temperature, mechanisms that keep the concentration of the internal fluids constant despite changes in the diet or fluid intake, mechanisms that compensate for blood loss and mechanisms that maintain a constant internal acid/base balance or pH.

3. List 3 ways in which animals keep their body temperature constant when the weather is hot.

Animals keep their body temperature constant when the weather is hot by keeping out of the sun, keeping activity to the minimum, sweating, panting and dilation of the surface blood vessels to increase heat loss to the environment.

4. How does the kidney compensate when an animal is deprived of water to drink?

The kidney compensates when an animal is deprived of water to drink through the action of the hormones antidiuretic hormone (ADH) and aldosterone, both of which act to increase the amount of water reabsorbed from the kidney tubule and increase the concentration of the urine produced. When the blood pressure decreases as occurs when fluid intake is insufficient, the reduced flow of blood through the glomerulus of the kidney tubule also reduces the amount of fluid filtered into the tubule so less urine is produced.

5. After moderate blood loss, several mechanisms come into play to increase blood pressure and make up blood volume. 3 of these mechanisms are:

After moderate blood loss, several mechanisms come into play to increase blood pressure and make up blood volume. These mechanisms include: thirst, constriction of blood vessels in the skin and kidneys, increasing heart rate, secretion of antidiuretic hormone and aldosterone, as well as drawing fluid from the tissues into the blood by increasing the osmotic pressure of the blood.

6. Describe how panting helps to reduce the acidity of the blood.

Panting helps to reduce the acidity of the blood by blowing out carbon dioxide. Carbon dioxide dissolved in the blood makes the blood acidic so removal of this carbon dioxide reduces the acidity of the blood.

Anatomy and Physiology of Animals/Glossary/Book version

A-B

Word	Meaning
A	
Abdomen	The part of the body below the diaphragm
Abomasum	The final compartment of the stomach of ruminants. This the 'true' stomach where muscular walls churn the food and gastric juice is secreted
Absorption	Passage of digested food from the gut into the blood
Accessory gland	A gland that produces secretions that make up the liquid portion of semen
Acetylcholine	A neurotransmitter released at a synapse
Acoustic	Relating to sound
Active transport	The movement of substances across a membrane against the concentration gradient. Requires energy
Adipose tissue	Connective tissue in which the cells are filled with fat or lipid
Adrenal cortex	Outer portion of adrenal gland
Adrenal medulla	Inner portion of adrenal gland
Albumin	The most common of the proteins in the plasma
Aldosterone	The hormone produced by the adrenal cortex
Alimentary	Concerning nutrition
Alimentary canal	The long canal from the mouth to the anus through which food passes as it is digested and absorbed
Alkaline	Containing few hydrogen ions. pH above 7
Alveolus	An air sac in the lung, where gas exchange takes place
Amino acids	Molecules containing nitrogen that are the building blocks of proteins
Amphibian	Vertebrate Class containing the frogs and toads
Amylases	Enzymes that split carbohydrates like starch and glycogen into monosaccharides like glucose
Anaemia	A condition involving a low number of red blood cells or haemoglobin in blood
Antagonistic muscles	A pair of muscles that work together such that as one contracts the other relaxes and vice versa.
Anterior	Nearer to the front of the body (usually used in human anatomy)
Anterior pituitary gland	Anterior portion of pituitary gland
Antibodies	Proteins made in response to a stimulating molecule called an antigen. The basis for the immune response
Anticoagulant	A substance that prevents blood clotting
Antidiuretic	A substance that inhibits urine production
Antidiuretic hormone	A hormone produced by posterior pituitary gland that stimulates water reabsorption from the kidney tubule
Antigens	A substance that stimulates the body to produce an antibody

Anus	The opening at the lower end of the rectum through which solid waste is eliminated.
Aorta	The main artery to body and head from heart
Apex	The pointed end of a cone shaped structure e.g. heart
Appendage	A structure attached to the body
Aqueous humor	The watery fluid that fills the anterior chamber of the eye
Arteriole	A small, almost microscopic, artery
Artery	A blood vessel that carries blood away from the heart
Articulation	The point of contact between bones. Where they move against each other
Appendage	A structure attached to the body
Aqueous humor	The watery fluid that fills the anterior chamber of the eye
Arteriole	A small, almost microscopic, artery
Artery	A blood vessel that carries blood away from the heart
Articulate	To move against each other - as of bones
Articulation	The point of contact between bones. Where they move against each other. A joint. Point of contact between 2 bones
Atlas	First cervical vertebra
Atom	A unit of matter that comprises a chemical element
Atrioventricular valve	A valve that prevents blood flow backwards from ventricle to atrium
Atrium (pl. atria)	One of two cranial chambers of heart
Auditory ossicle	One of 3 small bones in middle ear
Autonomic nervous system	The part of the vertebrate nervous system that innervates smooth and cardiac muscle and glandular tissues and governs involuntary actions. Consists of the sympathetic nervous system and the parasympathetic nervous system.
Axillary lymph node	A lymph node under junction of forelimb and body
Axis	The second cervical vertebra
Axon	A long extension from the neuron that carries nerve impulses away from the cell body
Ball and socket joint	A synovial joint where rounded end of one bone fits into cup-shaped depression of another
B	
Barb	The part of the feather that sticks out of the shaft
Barbules	The parts of a feather that grow out of the barbs. They have hooks and rolled edges to lock the barbs together
Basement membrane	The thin membrane between epidermis and dermis
Basophil	A white blood cell with granules in the cytoplasm
Biceps	The muscle that extends from the shoulder to the elbow responsible for flexing the forearm
Bilateral	Including both sides
Bile	An alkaline secretion from liver that helps break down fats into small droplets
Binocular vision	The placement of the eyes such that both see the same wide area but from slightly different angles
Binomial	The two-part Latinized name of a species, consisting of genus and species names
Blastocyst	A hollow ball of cells that develop from the fertilized ovum
Blind spot	The area of retina at end of optic nerve where there are no receptor cells

Blood	The fluid that circulates in the blood vessels
Blood pressure	The pressure of blood on the walls of the blood vessels
Body cavity	A space within the body that contains various organs
Bowman's capsule	The double walled globe at proximal end of nephron. Encloses glomerulus
Brain stem	The part of the brain just above the spinal cord. Contains the medulla oblongata
Breed	A race or variety
Bronchiole	A branch of the bronchi in the respiratory system
Bronchus	One of the large branches of the trachea
Buccal	To do with the mouth

C-D

Word	Meaning
C	
Callus	A thickening of the skin or growth of new bone tissue in and around a fracture
Canines	The long, cone-shaped teeth just behind the incisors
Carbohydrate	An organic compound containing carbon, hydrogen and oxygen. Made up of sugar subunits
Cardiac cycle	A complete heartbeat consisting of systole and diastole
Cardiac muscle	The muscle that makes up the wall of the heart. Striated branched fibres
Cardiovascular system	The body system comprising the heart, blood vessels and blood
Carnassial teeth	The modified premolars and molars in carnivores that slice against each other like scissors for shearing flesh and bone.
Carotid artery	The artery from aorta that supplies the head and brain
Carpal	A bone of the "wrist"
Cartilage	Dense connective tissue found at ends of long bones, in trachea, ear pinna. Also forms the skeleton of the foetus
Cataract	A condition in which the lens becomes cloudy resulting in blurred vision.
Caudal	Nearer to the tail than
Caudal vena cava	The large vein that collects blood from the body caudal to the heart
Cell	The basic structural and functional unit of all organisms
Cell division	The process by which a cell reproduces itself. Two types: mitosis and meiosis
Cell inclusion	A substance produced by cell that is free in cytoplasm i.e. not enclosed by a membrane
Cellular respiration	The chemical pathway that produces energy in the cell It consumes a fuel, generally glucose, in the presence of oxygen
Central nervous system	The part of the nervous system consisting of the brain and spinal cord
Cephalic	To do with the head
Cerebellum	The part of the vertebrate hindbrain located dorsally; functions in unconscious coordination of movement and balance
Cerebral cortex	The surface of the cerebrum; the largest and most complex part of the mammalian brain, containing sensory and motor nerve cell bodies of the cerebrum
Cerebrospinal fluid	The fluid that circulates around and within brain and spinal cord
Cerebrum	The dorsal portion of the brain composed of right and left hemispheres; the integrating center for memory, learning, emotions

Cervical vertebrae	The neck vertebrae
Cervix	The neck of the uterus
Chemoreceptor	A receptor that detects chemicals
Chorionic gonadotrophin	The hormone secreted by the placenta that prevents uterine contractions before labour and prepares the mammary glands for lactation
Choroid	The middle coat of the eyeball
Chromosome	One of the small dark staining bodies in the cell nucleus. Contains the DNA
Chyle	The milky fluid found in the lacteals of the small intestine
Chyme	The semi fluid mixture of partly digested food and digestive secretions in the stomach and small intestine
Cilium (pl. cilia)	A hair like process projecting from a cell. Used to move cell substances along the surface of the cell
Class	The taxonomic grouping of related, similar orders; category above order and below phylum
Clavicle	The collar bone
Clot	The process that changes liquid blood to a gelatinous mass
Coagulation	The process by which blood clots
Coccyx	The tail bones
Coccygeal vertebrae	The vertebrae of the tail
Cochlea	The coiled tube forming the portion of the inner ear that converts sound waves to nerve impulses
Collagen	A protein that is the main organic constituent of connective tissue
Colon	Part of the large intestine.
Colostrum	The first milk, it contains antibodies.
Common bile duct	The duct that carries both bile and pancreatic juice into the small intestine
Compact bone	Dense bone made up of Haversian systems
Conditioned Reflex	The response that is elicited by a stimulus after training has taken place
Condyle	A rounded protuberance at the ends of some bones where it forms an articulation with another bone
Cone	A light sensitive receptor in the retina that responds to colour
Congenital	Present at the time of birth
Conjunctiva	The delicate membrane covering the cornea of the eye
Connective tissue	One of the 4 basic tissue types of the body. Binds and supports. Consists of cells and fibres in a matrixs
Constipation	Decreased defecation due to decreased mobility of the intestines
Continuous breeding	When breeding continues throughout the year
Cornea	The transparent anterior layer of the eye through which the iris can be seen
Coronary artery	The artery that supplies the heart muscle
Corpus luteum	A yellow endocrine gland formed in the empty ovarian follicle after ovulation
Cortex	The outer layer of an organ
Costal	To do with a rib
Cowper's gland	One of the accessory glands of the male reproductive system
Cranial	Towards the head
Cranial nerve	One of the 12 nerves that leave the brain
Cranium	The brain case that surrounds and protects the brain

Crop	The bag-like structure at the base of the oesophagus in birds.In many birds it stores food before it enters the stomachA
Crop-milk	Secretion produced by glands in the wall of the crop of in pigeons and doves Parents regurgitate it to feed their young
Cross section	Crosswise slice of an animal or organ
Cryptorchidism	Undescended testes
Cutaneous	To do with the skin
Cytology	The study of cells
Cytosol	The semi fluid portion of the cytoplasm
D	
Dehydration	Excessive loss of water from the body or its parts
Denaturation	Disruption of the structure of a protein by heat, acids etc. to make it inactive
Dendrite	A nerve cell process that carries the nerve impulses towards the cell body
Dental formula	The formula that describes the numbers of the different kinds of teeth
Dentine	The tissue below the enamel in teeth
Dermis	The layer of dense connective tissue lying under the epidermis
Diabetes insipidus	The condition caused by under secretion of antidiuretic hormone (ADH). Symptom: excretion large amounts dilute urine
Diabetes mellitus	The condition caused by under secretion of insulin. Symptoms: raised blood glucose levels, glucose in urine
Diaphragm	The dome shaped skeletal muscle separating the thoracic from the abdominal cavities
Diaphysis	The shaft of a long bone
Diarrhoea	Frequent defecation of liquid faeces
Diastema	The space in the jaw in animals that have no (or reduced) canines
Diastole	The phase of the heartbeat involving the relaxation of the ventricles
Diastolic blood pressure	Blood pressure in the arteries between the passage of the pulses
Diffusion	A passive process of movement of molecules from a region of high concentration to one of low concentration
Digestion	The mechanical and physical breakdown of food
Digitigrade locomotion	Locomotion on the "fingers" as in cats and dogs
Dilate	To expand or swell
Diploid	Having a double set of chromosomes one maternal, one paternal
Directional terms	Terms that describe the locations of structures in relation to other structures or locations in the body
Disaccharides	Double sugar, consisting of two joined monosaccharides
Distal	Farther away from the trunk of the body or point of origin
Diuretic	A chemical that reduces Antidiuretic hormone production and increases urine volume
Dorsal	Nearer the back of the animal than
Duodenum	First part of the small intestine

E-F

Word	Meaning
E	
Echolocation	The use of high frequency sound like sonar and radar by animals (i.e. whales and bats) to locate objects in the surrounding environment
Effector	A muscle or gland that responds to a motor neuron impulse
Egestion	The elimination of indigestible waste products from the body
Electrolyte	A compound that separates into charged particles or ions
Electron microscope	A microscope that focuses an electron beam through a specimen, resulting in resolving power a thousandfold greater than that of a light microscope
Element	Any substance that cannot be broken down to any other substance
Embryo	The young of any organism in an early stage of development
Emulsification	The breakdown of large fat particles to smaller ones in the presence of bile
Enamel	The hard white substance covering the crown of teeth
Endocrine gland	A ductless gland that secretes hormones into the blood
Endometrium	The inner lining of the uterus
Endoplasmic reticulum	The network of membranous channels running through the cytoplasm of cells
Endothelium	The layer of squamous epithelium that lines blood vessels
Enzyme	A substance that increases the speed of a chemical reaction
Eosinophil	A white blood cell with granules in the cytoplasm
Epidermis	The thin outer layer of the skin
Epididymis	The organ composed of convoluted tubules that lies on the border of the testis Where sperm mature
Epiglottis	The cartilage on the top of the larynx that closes the windpipe during swallowing
Epiphyseal line	The remnant of epiphyseal plate at end of long bone
Epiphyseal plate	The cartilaginous plate at the end of a long bone where bone growth occurs
Epiphysis	The end of a long bone
Epithelial tissue	Tissue that forms outer part of skin, lines blood vessels, hollow organs and passages in the body
Erythrocyte	A red blood cell
Essential amino acids	The 10 amino acids that can not be made by animals and must be acquired in the diet
Eustachian tube	The passage connecting middle ear to pharynx. Equalises air pressure in middle and outer ear
Evolution	All the changes that have transformed life on Earth from its earliest beginnings to the diversity that characterizes it today
Excretion	To cast out material from the body, cell or tissue
Exocrine gland	A gland that secretes substances into a duct
Exocytosis	The discharge of substances through the plasma membrane
Expiration	Breathing out
Extension	Bending of a joint so that the angle between the bones increases
Extracellular fluid	Fluid outside body cells
F	
Facilitated diffusion	Diffusion across a membrane using a carrier substance

Fallopian tube	A slender tube through which eggs pass from an ovary to the uterus
Fats	Biological compounds consisting of three fatty acids linked to one glycerol molecule
Feedback system	The sequence of events where information about the status of a situation is continually fed back to the central control region
Femur	The long bone between the pelvis and the knee
Fertilisation	Penetration of ovum by sperm and union of nuclei
Fetlock	The joint between the metacarpals or metatarsals and the phalanges in horse
Fibrin	The insoluble protein formed from fibrinogen
Fibrinogen	The protein in blood plasma essential for blood clotting
Fibula	The lateral bone of the lower hind limb
Filtrate	The fluid produced by filtration of blood in the nephron
Flagellum	A long hair like process e.g. tail of sperm
Flexion	The movement involving decreasing the angle between two bones
Fluoroxylate	An anticoagulant used for biochemical tests for glucose
Foetus	Later stage of development of a young animal
Follicle	The cavity surrounding the developing ovum
Follicle stimulating hormone (FSH)	Hormone secreted by anterior pituitary gland. Stimulates development of ovarian follicle
Foramen	A hole in a bone for passage of vessels or nerves
Foramen magnum	The hole at the base of the skull for passage of the spinal cord
Fossa	A furrow or shallow depression in a bone
Fovea	The area of the retina of greatest concentration of cone cells. Area of sharpest vision
Functional caecum	The enlarged large intestine and caecum occupied by cellulose digesting micro-organisms

G-H

Word	Meaning
G	
Gall bladder	The small pouch that stores bile
Gamete	A reproductive cell - sperm or ovum
Ganglion	A group of nerve cells outside central nervous system
Gas exchange	The process in which oxygen from inhaled air is transferred into the blood and carbon dioxide from the blood is transferred into the alveoli
Gastric juice	The digestive secretion produced by glands in the wall of the stomach
Gene	A biological unit of heredity
Gestation	The period of foetal development inside the uterus
Girdle	An encircling or arching arrangement of bones
Gizzard	The second part of the stomach of birds. In seed eating birds it contains pebbles and its muscular walls help grind the food
Gland	A collection of cells that secrete substances
Gliding joint	A synovial joint with flat articulating surfaces that permits limited movements e.g. between carpals and tarsals

Glomerular capsule	See Bowman's capsule
Glomerulus	Tuft of capillaries surrounded by the Bowman's capsule in nephron
Glottis	Vocal cords
Glucose	The smallest sugar. Major energy source for all cells
Glycerol	A molecule that combines with three fatty acid molecules to form a fat or oil
Glycogen	A highly branched polymer of glucose. Energy store in body
Goitre	A condition involving enlargement of thyroid gland
Golgi complex apparatus	A cell organelle concerned with packaging, processing and secretion of organic molecules
Gonads	The ovary and testes
Graafian follicle	The mature ovarian follicle
Grey matter	Area of the nervous system consisting of cell bodies
Growth hormone	A hormone secreted by the anterior pituitary gland. Stimulates growth, particularly of the skeleton
H	
Haematocrit	The percentage of blood made up of red blood cells. Also called packed cell volume (PCV)
Haematuria	Urine that contains red blood cells
Haemoglobin	Pigment containing iron in red blood cells that allows them to carry oxygen
Haemolysis	The escape of haemoglobin from a red blood cell
Haemorrhage	Bleeding
Haploid	Having half the normal number of chromosomes, produced by meiosis
Haversian canal	The canal down centre of a Haversian system
Haversian system	The columns of boney tissue that make up compact bone
Heparin	A naturally occurring anticoagulant. Also used in laboratory tests for heavy metals
Hepatic	To do with the liver
Hepatic portal vessel	The blood vessel that carries blood from the intestines to the liver
Hinge joint	A synovial joint that allows movement in only one plane e.g. elbow
Histamine	A substance secreted from white cells and platelets that is involved in the inflammatory response
Hock	The joint (between the tarsals and metatarsals
Homoiothermic	'Warm-blooded' animals that regulate their body temperature
Hormone	A secretion from an endocrine gland
Humerus	The bone of the upper forearm between the scapula and the radius and ulna
Hyperglycemia	Elevated blood glucose level
Hypertension	High blood pressure
Hyperthermia	High body temperature
Hypertonic	Having an osmotic pressure higher than a solution with which it is compared
Hypotension	Low blood pressure
Hypotonic	Having an osmotic pressure lower than a solution with which it is compared

I-J

Word	Meaning
I	
Ileum	The terminal part of the small intestine
Immunity	Being resistant to injury or invasion by microorganisms
Implantation	The attachment of blastocyst to lining of uterus
Impotence	The inability to copulate
Incisors	The chisel-shaped 'biting off' teeth at the front of the mouth
Induced ovulation	When ovulation is stimulated by mating as in cat and rabbit
Inferior	Towards the lower part of the body. Not used in animals except, perhaps, higher apes
Infertility	The inability to conceive or cause conception
Inflammation	A localised protective response to tissue injury
Ingestion	The taking in of food, liquids etc.
Inguinal	To do with the groin
Inorganic	Compounds that lack carbon
Insertion	The attachment of a muscle tendon to a bone that moves
Inspiration	Breathing in
Insulin	A hormone produced by the pancreas. Decreases blood glucose levels
Intercostal muscles	The muscles between the ribs.
Internal	Away from the surface of the body
Interstitial fluid	Extracellular fluid surrounding the cells
Intervertebral disc	A pad of cartilage between the vertebrae
Intestinal juice	Digestive secretion produced by glands in the lining of the small intestine
Intracellular fluid	Fluid within the cells
Invertebrates	Animals that do not posses a backbone or vertebral column
Ion	A charged particle
Isotonic	Having an osmotic pressure equal to that of a solution with which it is compared
J	
Jejunum	The middle portion of the small intestine

K-L

Word	Meaning
K	
Keel	The breast bone in birds
Keratin	A protein found in epidermis, hair, feathers, hoofs etc.
Kidney	The organ that produces urine
L	
Lachrymal gland	The tear gland of the eye
Lacteal	A lymphatic vessel within the villi of the small intestine
Lacuna	A small hollow space
Lamellae	Concentric rings of hard calcified material found in compact bone
Large intestine	Part of the gut consisting of the colon, caecum, rectum and anal canal
Larynx	The voice box
Lateral	Away from the midline
Lens	Transparent part of the eye that helps focus light rays on the retina
Leukocyte	A white blood cell
Ligament	Dense connective tissue that attaches bone to bone
Lipase	Digestive enzyme that breaks down fats (lipids)
Lipid	Fat
Liver	The large organ caudal to the diaphragm
Longitudinal	Lengthwise slice of an animal or organ
Lordosis response	Standing firm to pressure on the loin region
Lumbar	Loin region of the back
Lumen	A space within an artery, vein, intestine or tube
Lung	The organs of respiration
Luteinising hormone	The hormone from the anterior pituitary gland that stimulates ovulation and development of corpus luteum
Lymph	Tissue fluid that has entered the lymphatic system
Lymph node	A structure that filters lymph and produces lymphocytes
Lymphatic capillary	The closed ended microscopic vessel that collects lymph in tissues
Lymphatic tissue	Specialised tissue that contains large numbers of lymphocytes
Lymphatic vessel	A large vessel that carries lymph
Lymphocyte	A white blood cell associated with the immune response
Lysosome	A cell organelle that contains digestive enzymes

M-N

Word	Meaning
M	
Macrophage	A large phagocytic cell present in many tissues
Mammary gland	The milk producing gland
Mandible	The bone of the lower jaw
Marrow	The soft sponge like material in the cavities of bone
Matrix	The substance of a tissue in which the more specialised structures are embedded
Maxilla	The bone of the upper jaw
Medial	Towards the midline
Mediastinum	The tissue that separates the two sides of the lung
Medulla	Inner part of an organ
Medulla oblongata	The part of the brain stem or hind brain
Meiosis	The type of cell division for production of gametes. Halves the number of chromosomes
Melanin	The dark pigment in the skin and hair
Melatonin	The hormone produced by the pineal gland
Membrane	A thin, flexible sheet of tissue
Meninges	The membranes covering the brain and spinal cord
Mesentery	The membrane attaching the small intestine to the abdominal wall
Metacarpals	The bones of the "hand"
Metastasis	The distant spread of disease especially a malignant tumour from its site of origin
Metatarsals	The five bones of the foot that connect the "ankle" to the toes
Microfilaments	A solid contracting strand in the cytoplasm of cells that brings about cell contraction.
Microtubule	A hollow rod of protein in the cytoplasm of all eukaryotic cells and in cilia, flagella, and the cytoskeleton
Microvilli	The microscopic fingerlike projections from the membrane of the cells covering the villi of the small intestine
Middle ear	The cavity in the skull between the eardrum and inner ear housing the auditory ossicles
Milk teeth	The first set of teeth in a young animal
Minute volume	The volume of air inspired or expired during a minute of normal tidal breathing
Mitochondrion	The organelle in cell cytoplasm that produces energy
Mitosis	The cell division for growth and repair. Produces 2 cells identical to parent and each othe
Molars	The more posterior cheek teeth
Monocyte	The largest leukocyte. It is phagocytic and has no granules in the cytoplasm
Monosaccharide	The simplest carbohydrate. Also known as simple sugar
Morula	The solid mass of cells produced by successive divisions of the fertilized ovum
Mucus	A thick fluid secretion
Myelin	The fatty insulating coating to an axon of a neuron
N	
Nasal cavity	The space just inside the nostril
Negative feedback	Control in which the stimulus initiates actions that reverse or reduce the stimulus

Nephron	The functional unit of the kidney
Nerve	A bundle of nerve fibres
Nerve impulse	The nerve "current' that passes along a neuron
Neuron	A nerve cell
Neurotransmitter	Molecules released at a synapse to transmit the nerve impulse from one neuron to the next
Neutral fat	A fat or triglyceride. Biological compound consisting of three fatty acids linked to one glycerol molecule
Neutrophil	White blood cell with granules in the cytoplasm involved in phagocytosis
Nictitating membrane	The third eyelid in the cat, tuatara and crocodiles
Normal saline	A 0.9% solution of sodium chloride
Nuclear membrane	The double layered membrane that surrounds the nucleus
Nucleolus	The spherical body within the nucleus, containing RNA
Nucleus	The spherical or oval body in the cell that contains the DNA
Nutrient	A chemical substance in food that provides energy or assists various body processes

O-P

Word	Meaning
O	
Excessive accumulation of fluid in the body tissues	
Oesophagus	The hollow muscular tube connecting the pharynx with stomach
The female sex hormone produced by ovaries	
Olfactory	To do with smell
Omasum	Part of the modified stomach of ruminants with a folded inner surface
Open rooted teeth	Teeth in which the root opening remains wide. They grow continuously e.g. the incisors of rabbits and rats
Optic Nerve	The nerve carrying impulses from the retina of the eye to the brain
Orbit	The bony cavity in the skull that holds the eyeball
Organ	A structure with a specific function
Organelle	A structure in the cell with a specific function
Organic	A compound that contains carbon and hydrogen e.g. carbohydrates, lipids and proteins
Organism	A living form. One individual
Origin	The attachment of a muscle to a bone that does not move
Osmosis	The movement of water molecules across a semi permeable membrane from an area of high water concentration to an area of low water concentration
Osmotic pressure	The pressure required to prevent water moving across a semi permeable membrane by osmosis
Ossicle	A small bone
Ossification	The formation of bone
Otolith	A particle of calcium carbonate embedded in the membrane of the otolith organ of the inner ear
Oval window	The small opening between the middle and inner ear

Ovarian cycle	The series of events in the ovary associated with the maturation of the ovum
Ovarian follicle	The developing ovum with the epithelial tissues surrounding it
Ovary	The female gonad that produces ova
Ovulation	The release of the ovum from the mature follicle of the ovary
Ovum	The egg cell (plural: ova)
Oxyhaemoglobin	Haemoglobin combined with oxygen
Oxytocin	The hormone from the posterior pituitary gland. Stimulates milk "let down"
P	
Palate	The roof of the mouth
Palmar	The "walking" surface of the front paw
Pancreas	The organ lying along the caudal margin of the stomach. Has endocrine and exocrine functions
Pancreatic juice	The digestive secretion produced by the pancreas
Parasympathetic division	One of the two parts of the autonomic nervous system. Concerned with normal "at rest" activities
Parathyroid gland	One of four small endocrine glands on the dorsal surface of the thyroid gland
Parathyroid hormone	The hormone secreted from the parathyroid gland
Parotid gland	One of the paired salivary glands ventral to the ear
Parturition	The act of giving birth
Patella	The kneecap
Pathogen	A disease-producing organism
Pectoral	To do with the chest or breast
Pelvic cavity	The caudal portion of the abdominal cavity. Contains the bladder, colon and reproductive structures
Pelvic girdle	The bony structure formed by the hip bones, sacrum and coccygeal bones
Pelvis	The structure formed by the two hip bones, sacrum and coccyx
Pepsin	A protein digesting enzyme secreted by the stomach wall
Pericardial cavity	The small cavity between the two layers of the pericardial membranes
Pericardium	The membrane that encloses the heart
Periosteum	The tough connective tissue covering of a bone
Peripheral	Located on the outer part of the body
Peripheral nervous system	The part of the nervous system composed of the cranial and spinal nerves
Peristalsis	The successive muscular contractions along the wall of the gut
Peritoneum	The membrane that lines the abdominal cavity and covers the abdominal organ
Permanent teeth	The second set of teeth that persist through life
Peyer's Patches	Large clusters of lymph nodules found in the wall of the small intestine
pH	A symbol that indicates the acidity or alkalinity of a solution
Phagocytosis	The process by which cells ingest particles and bacteria
Phalanges	The bones of the "fingers" and "toes"
Pharynx	The throat
Phospholipid bilayer	The arrangement of phospholipids molecules in two layers
Phospholipids	Molecules that make up the double layer of biological membranes

Photoreceptor	A receptor that detects light
Photosynthesis	The making of organic molecules by plants using energy from the sun
Physiology	The science that deals with the functions of an organism and its parts
Pineal gland	The gland situated in the brain that secretes melatoni
Pinna	The projecting part of the external ear
Pinocytosis	The process by which cells ingest liquid
Pituitary gland	The endocrine gland lying under the caudal surface of the brain attached to the hypothalamus by a stalk
Pivot joint	A synovial joint where a peg of bone articulates with a ring of bone as in the joint between the atlas and axis
Placenta	The special structure through which the exchange of materials between the foetus and mother occurs
Plantar	The "walking" surface of the hind paw
Plantigrade locomotion	Locomotion involving placing the whole surface of the foot on the ground as in humans and bears
Plasma	The fluid that surrounds the blood cells
Plasma membrane	The outer membrane surrounding the cell
Platelets	Cell fragments in the blood essential for clotting
Pleura	Membranes that cover the lungs and line the walls of the chest and diaphragm
Pleural cavity	The space between the two layers of the pleura
Plexus	A network of nerves
Poikilothermic	'Cold-blooded' animals whose body temperature varies, to a large extent depending on the environment
Polysaccharides	A carbohydrate formed from up to a thousand monosaccharides
Preen	To clean, straighten and fluff feathers
Premolars	The more anterior cheek teeth
Progesterone	The hormone produced by the corpus luteum
Prolactin	A hormone produced by the anterior pituitary gland
Prostate gland	The gland caudal to bladder in males
Proteases	Enzymes that split proteins into amino acids
Protein	An organic compound consisting of carbon, hydrogen, oxygen and nitrogen. Made up of amino acids
Proximal	Nearer to the body or to the point of origin
Pulmonary	To do with the lungs
Pulp cavity	The cavity within the crown and neck of a toot
Pulse	The series of waves of high pressure blood passing along an artery
Pupil	The hole in the centre of the iris of the eye
Pus	Dead white blood cells
Pyloric sphincter	The ring of smooth muscle between the stomach and the small intestine

Q,R,S

Word	Meaning
R	
Radius	The shorter bone of the forelimb between the humerus and the "wrist"
Receptor	A specialized cell that responds to specific sensory stimuli such as touch,pressure, light etc.
Red marrow	Bone marrow found in the spaces of spongy bone.Makes red blood cells
Reflex	A fast automatic response to a stimulus
Reflex arc	Consists of receptor, sensory, relay and motor neurons and effector
Refraction	Bending of light as it passes from one medium to another
Relaxin	The hormone secreted by the placenta and ovaries that eases the joint between the right and left pelvis and dilates the cervix for birth
Renal	To do with the kidney
Renal pelvis	The cavity in the centre of the kidney
Renal pyramid	A cone shaped structure in kidney medulla
Renal system	The body system involving the kidneys
Reticulum	The part of the modified stomach of ruminants with honeycomb of raised folds on its inner surface
Retina	The inner coat of the eyeball. Nerve calls here (rods and cones} respond to light ray
Ribosome	The organelle in the cell that makes proteins
Rickets	A bone disorder caused by inadequate vitamin D
Rod	The photoreceptor in the retina, specialized for vision in dim light
Rostral	Towards the muzzle
Rumen	The first and largest compartment of the modified stomach of ruminants.It houses the microorganisms
Ruminant	An animal with a rumen e.g. sheep, cow, camel
Rumination	Chewing the "cud"
S	
Sacrum	The triangular bone formed from fused sacral vertebrae.Located between the two hipbones
Sagittal plane	Plane that divides the body into left and right portions
Sagittal section	Lengthwise slice of an animal or organ
Saliva	The secretion from the salivary glands
Salivary amylase	The starch digesting enzyme in saliva
Saturated fat	A fat containing saturated fatty acids
Scapula	The shoulder blade
Sciatic nerve	The large nerve that passes down the hind leg
Sclera	The fibrous outer coat of eyeball
Seasonal breeding	Breeding confined to certain seasons of the year
Sebaceous gland	An exocrine gland in the dermis of the skin associated with a hair follicle
Sebum	The waxy secretion from a sebaceous gland
Secondary sex characteristic	A characteristic that develops at sexual maturity. e.g. large body size of males, manes in lions
Secretion	The production or release of a fluid from a gland

Semen	The fluid discharged at ejaculation of male. Consists of sperm and fluid
Semicircular canals	The membranous fluid filled canals containing receptors for equilibrium
Semilunar valve	The valve guarding the entrance to the aorta or the pulmonary artery
Seminal vesicle	A gland that secretes a component of semen
Seminiferous tubule	The tightly coiled duct in the testis where sperm are produced
Semi-permeable membrane	A membrane that allows some substances to cross more easily than others
Sensory neuron	A neuron that carries a nerve impulse towards the central nervous system
Serum	Plasma minus its clotting proteins
Sesamoid bones	Small bones usually found in tendons
Shock	Reduced cardiac output resulting in failure to deliver adequate oxygen and nutrients to the body
Shoulder	The synovial joint where the humerus joins the scapula
Sinus	An air cavity in a bone especially in the bones of the face or skull
Skeletal muscle	Tissue specialized for contraction with striated fibres. Attached to the bones of the skeleton
Skull	The skeleton of the head
Small intestine	The long tube of the gut that begins at the stomach and ends at the large intestine
Smooth muscle	Tissue specialized for contraction with spindle shaped non striated fibres
Soft palate	The posterior portion of the roof of the mouth
Solution	One or more substances dissolved in a liquid
Specific gravity	A measure of the density of a liquid or solid, as compared with that of water.
Sperm duct	The tube that carries sperm from the epididymis to the urethra. Also called the vas deferens
Spermatic cord	The structure in the male reproductive system attached to the testis that carries the vas deferens, arteries, veins, etc.
Spermatozoon	A mature sperm cell
Sphincter	A ring-like muscle that controls movement along a body passage or orifice
Spinal cord	The mass of nerve tissue in the vertebral column
Spinal nerve	One of the nerves that originate in the spinal cord
Spleen	The large lymphatic organ near the stomach that stores blood and produces lymphocytes
Spongy bone	The inner layer of bone; found at the ends of long bones less dense than compact bone
Squamous	Scale like
Starch	The storage polysaccharide in plants consisting of many glucose molecules
Sterile	Free from any living micro organisms
Sternum	The breastbone
Stifle	The joint between the femur and the tibia on the hind leg
Stimulus	Any change in the environment capable of initiating a nerve impulse
Stomach	The large baglike part of the gut between the oesophagus and the small intestine
Striated muscle	Striped or skeletal muscle
Subcutaneous	Beneath the skin
Submandibular gland	The salivary gland beneath the tongue
Substrate	A substance on which an enzyme acts
Sulcus	A groove or depression between the convolutions of the brain

Superficial	Nearer to the surface of
Suture	An immoveable joint in the skull
Sympathetic division	One of the two subdivisions of the autonomic nervous system concerned with reacting to emergency situations
Synapse	The junction between two neurons
Synovial joint	A fully moveable joint
System	An association of organs that have a common function, e.g. digestive system, respiratory system
Systemic circulation	The blood circulation from the left ventricl through the aorta to all the organs of the body and back to the heart
Systole	The phase of the heartbeat involving contraction of the ventricles
Systolic blood pressure	The blood pressure during passage of the pulse
Synapse	The junction between two neurons
Synovial joint	A fully moveable joint

T,U,V,W,X,Y,Z

Word	Meaning
T	
Target cell	A cell whose activity is affected by a particular hormone
Tarsals	The bones of the "ankle"
Tendons	A tough cord of fibrous connective tissue that connects muscles to bones
Testis	The male gonad that produces sperm
Testosterone	The hormone produced by the cells between the seminiferous tubules of the testis
Thoracic cavity	The chest cavity that contains the heart and lungs
Thorax	The part of the body between the neck and the diaphragm
Thymus gland	The organ dorsal to the sternum that is essential to the immune response
Thyroid gland	The endocrine gland with lobes on either side of the trachea
Thyroxine	The hormone secreted by the thyroid gland
Tibia	The medial bone of the lower hind limb
Tidal breathing	Normal at rest breathing
Tidal volume	The volume of air breathed in or out in any one "at rest" breath
Tissue	A group of similar cells
Tissue fluid	Plasma that has left the capillaries and flowed into the spaces between the cells of the tissues; also known as intercellular fluid or interstitial fluid
Total lung capacity	The sum of the tidal volume, inspiratory reserve, expiratory reserve and residual volume of the lungs
Trachea	The windpipe
Transverse	A crosswise slice of an animal or organ
Triceps	The muscle that extends from the shoulder to the elbow responsible for extending the forearm
Triglycerides	A biological compound consisting of three fatty acids linked to one glycerol molecule. A fat
Trunk	The part of the body to which the fore and hind limbs are attached
Tympanic membrane	The thin transparent membrane of connective tissue between the external ear, canal and the middle ear. Also called the eardrum

U	
Ulna	The longer bone of the forelimb between the humerus and the "wrist"
Umbilical cord	The cord containing arteries and vein that attaches the foetus to the placenta
Unguligrade locomotion	Locomotion on the "fingernails" as in horses and pigs
Urea	The soluble excretory product produced when excess amino acids (from proteins) are broken down by the body
Ureter	One of two tubes that connect the kidney with the bladder
Urethra	The duct from the bladder to the exterior of the body
Uric acid	An insoluble excretory product produced when excess amino acids(from proteins) are broken down by the body
Urinalysis	The analysis of urine
Urine	The fluid produced by the kidneys
Uterus	The hollow muscular organ in females where the foetus develops
V	
Vagina	The muscular, tubular organ in the female where sperm are deposited during copulation
Vagus nerve	The cranial nerve that controls the muscles that bring about swallowing,the muscles of the heart, airways, lungs, stomach and intestines
Vane	The flat part of a feather emerging from the shaft; there are two vanes per feather
Vas deferens	The duct that conducts the sperm from the epididymis to the urethra
Vascular	To do with blood
Vasoconstriction	The decrease in size of the channel down a blood vessel
Vaso dilation	The increase in size of the channel down a blood vessel
Vein	A blood vessel that carries blood towards the heart
Velvet	The tissue layer that covers antlers
Vena cava	One of two large blood vessels that return blood to the heart
Ventral	Nearer the belly of the animal than
Ventricles	The caudal chambers of the heart
Venule	A small vein
Vertebral canal	The channel that encloses and protects the spinal cord
Vertebrates	Animals that have a backbone or vertebral column
Vesicles	Small, intracellular membrane-bound sac
Vestibular organ	The organ of balance – semicircular canals and otolith organ
Villus (pl. villi)	A projection from the lining of the small intestine to help absorb digested food molecules
Viscera	The organs in the abdominal and pelvic cavities
Visceral skeleton	Bones formed in the organs of the body
Viscosity	The thickness or stickiness of a liquid
Vital capacity	The sum of the inspiratory and expiratory reserve volumes and the tidal volume
Vital capacity	The volume of the air expired when a maximum expiration follows a maximum inspiration
Vitamin	An organic molecule necessary in minute quantities for the proper functioning of the chemical processes in the body
Vitreous Humor	The fluid in the posterior chamber of the eye
W	

White matter	Masses of myelinated axons located in the brain and spinal cord
Y	
Yellow marrow	Bone marrow that is yellow with fat; found at the ends of long bones
Z	
Zona pellucida	The tough layer surrounding the ovum
Zygote	Single cell resulting from the union of the sperm and egg

Article Sources and Contributors

Anatomy and Physiology of Animals *Source*: http://en.wikibooks.org/w/index.php?oldid=2060066 *Contributors*: -

Anatomy and Physiology of Animals/Preface *Source*: http://en.wikibooks.org/w/index.php?oldid=1530283 *Contributors*: -

Anatomy and Physiology of Animals/The Author *Source*: http://en.wikibooks.org/w/index.php?oldid=1530316 *Contributors*: -

Anatomy and Physiology of Animals/Acknowledgements *Source*: http://en.wikibooks.org/w/index.php?oldid=1530134 *Contributors*: -

Anatomy and Physiology of Animals/Table of contents *Source*: http://en.wikibooks.org/w/index.php?oldid=1530315 *Contributors*: -

Anatomy and Physiology of Animals/Chemicals *Source*: http://en.wikibooks.org/w/index.php?oldid=2054886 *Contributors*: -

Anatomy and Physiology of Animals/Chemicals/Test Yourself Answers *Source*: http://en.wikibooks.org/w/index.php?oldid=1530206 *Contributors*: -

Anatomy and Physiology of Animals/Classification *Source*: http://en.wikibooks.org/w/index.php?oldid=2122406 *Contributors*: -

Anatomy and Physiology of Animals/Classification/Test Yourself Answers *Source*: http://en.wikibooks.org/w/index.php?oldid=1530212 *Contributors*: -

Anatomy and Physiology of Animals/The Cell *Source*: http://en.wikibooks.org/w/index.php?oldid=2053640 *Contributors*: -

Anatomy and Physiology of Animals/The Cell/Test Yourself Answers *Source*: http://en.wikibooks.org/w/index.php?oldid=1530344 *Contributors*: -

Anatomy and Physiology of Animals/Body Organisation *Source*: http://en.wikibooks.org/w/index.php?oldid=2095976 *Contributors*: -

Anatomy and Physiology of Animals/Body Organisation/Test Yourself Answers *Source*: http://en.wikibooks.org/w/index.php?oldid=1530165 *Contributors*: -

Anatomy and Physiology of Animals/The Skin *Source*: http://en.wikibooks.org/w/index.php?oldid=2105544 *Contributors*: -

Anatomy and Physiology of Animals/The Skin/Test Yourself Answers *Source*: http://en.wikibooks.org/w/index.php?oldid=1530453 *Contributors*: -

Anatomy and Physiology of Animals/The Skeleton *Source*: http://en.wikibooks.org/w/index.php?oldid=1984319 *Contributors*: -

Anatomy and Physiology of Animals/The Skeleton/Test Yourself Answers *Source*: http://en.wikibooks.org/w/index.php?oldid=1530432 *Contributors*: -

Anatomy and Physiology of Animals/Muscles *Source*: http://en.wikibooks.org/w/index.php?oldid=2126420 *Contributors*: -

Anatomy and Physiology of Animals/Muscles/Test Yourself Answers *Source*: http://en.wikibooks.org/w/index.php?oldid=1530260 *Contributors*: -

Anatomy and Physiology of Animals/Cardiovascular System *Source*: http://en.wikibooks.org/w/index.php?oldid=1689835 *Contributors*: -

Anatomy and Physiology of Animals/Cardiovascular System/Blood *Source*: http://en.wikibooks.org/w/index.php?oldid=2114884 *Contributors*: -

Anatomy and Physiology of Animals/Cardiovascular System/Blood/Test Yourself Answers *Source*: http://en.wikibooks.org/w/index.php?oldid=1530174 *Contributors*: -

Anatomy and Physiology of Animals/Cardiovascular System/The Heart *Source*: http://en.wikibooks.org/w/index.php?oldid=2054449 *Contributors*: -

Anatomy and Physiology of Animals/Cardiovascular System/The Heart/Test Yourself Answers *Source*: http://en.wikibooks.org/w/index.php?oldid=1530192 *Contributors*: -

Anatomy and Physiology of Animals/Cardiovascular System/Blood circulation *Source*: http://en.wikibooks.org/w/index.php?oldid=2079865 *Contributors*: -

Anatomy and Physiology of Animals/Cardiovascular System/Blood circulation/Test Yourself Answers *Source*: http://en.wikibooks.org/w/index.php?oldid=1530184 *Contributors*: -

Anatomy and Physiology of Animals/Respiratory System *Source*: http://en.wikibooks.org/w/index.php?oldid=1757107 *Contributors*: -

Anatomy and Physiology of Animals/Respiratory System/Test Yourself Answers *Source*: http://en.wikibooks.org/w/index.php?oldid=1530314 *Contributors*: -

Anatomy and Physiology of Animals/Lymphatic System *Source*: http://en.wikibooks.org/w/index.php?oldid=2054506 *Contributors*: -

Anatomy and Physiology of Animals/Lymphatic System/Test Yourself Answers *Source*: http://en.wikibooks.org/w/index.php?oldid=1530253 *Contributors*: -

Anatomy and Physiology of Animals/The Gut and Digestion *Source*: http://en.wikibooks.org/w/index.php?oldid=2053641 *Contributors*: -

Anatomy and Physiology of Animals/The Gut and Digestion/Test Yourself Answers *Source*: http://en.wikibooks.org/w/index.php?oldid=1530371 *Contributors*: -

Anatomy and Physiology of Animals/Urinary System *Source*: http://en.wikibooks.org/w/index.php?oldid=2159492 *Contributors*: -

Anatomy and Physiology of Animals/Urinary System/Test Yourself Answers *Source*: http://en.wikibooks.org/w/index.php?oldid=1530471 *Contributors*: -

Anatomy and Physiology of Animals/Reproductive System *Source*: http://en.wikibooks.org/w/index.php?oldid=2071865 *Contributors*: -

Anatomy and Physiology of Animals/Reproductive System/Test Yourself Answers *Source*: http://en.wikibooks.org/w/index.php?oldid=1530303 *Contributors*: -

Anatomy and Physiology of Animals/Nervous System *Source*: http://en.wikibooks.org/w/index.php?oldid=2124647 *Contributors*: -

Anatomy and Physiology of Animals/Nervous System/Test Yourself Answers *Source*: http://en.wikibooks.org/w/index.php?oldid=1530279 *Contributors*: -

Anatomy and Physiology of Animals/The Senses *Source*: http://en.wikibooks.org/w/index.php?oldid=2055703 *Contributors*: -

Anatomy and Physiology of Animals/The Senses/Senses Test Yourself Answers *Source*: http://en.wikibooks.org/w/index.php?oldid=1530395 *Contributors*: -

Anatomy and Physiology of Animals/Endocrine System *Source*: http://en.wikibooks.org/w/index.php?oldid=2079497 *Contributors*: -

Anatomy and Physiology of Animals/Endocrine System/Test Yourself Answers *Source*: http://en.wikibooks.org/w/index.php?oldid=1598945 *Contributors*: -

Anatomy and Physiology of Animals/Glossary/Book version *Source*: http://en.wikibooks.org/w/index.php?oldid=2053393 *Contributors*: -

Image Sources, Licenses and Contributors

was Sunshineconnelly at en.wikibooks

File:Anatomy and physiology of animals stratified squamous epithelium.jpg *Source*: http://en.wikibooks.org/w/index.php?title=File:Anatomy_and_physiology_of_animals_stratified_squamous_epithelium.jpg *License*: Creative Commons Attribution 2.5 *Contributors*: Original uploader was Sunshineconnelly at en.wikibooks

File:Anatomy and physiology of animals loose connective tissue.jpg *Source*: http://en.wikibooks.org/w/index.php?title=File:Anatomy_and_physiology_of_animals_loose_connective_tissue.jpg *License*: Creative Commons Attribution 2.5 *Contributors*: Original uploader was Sunshineconnelly at en.wikibooks

File:Anatomy and Physiology of animals cartilage.jpg *Source*: http://en.wikibooks.org/w/index.php?title=File:Anatomy_and_Physiology_of_animals_cartilage.jpg *License*: Creative Commons Attribution 2.5 *Contributors*: Original uploader was Sunshineconnelly at en.wikibooks

File:Anatomy and physiology of animals smooth muscle fibres.jpg *Source*: http://en.wikibooks.org/w/index.php?title=File:Anatomy_and_physiology_of_animals_smooth_muscle_fibres.jpg *License*: Creative Commons Attribution 2.5 *Contributors*: Original uploader was Sunshineconnelly at en.wikibooks

File:Anatomy and physiology of animals skeletal muscle fibres.jpg *Source*: http://en.wikibooks.org/w/index.php?title=File:Anatomy_and_physiology_of_animals_skeletal_muscle_fibres.jpg *License*: Creative Commons Attribution 2.5 *Contributors*: Original uploader was Sunshineconnelly at en.wikibooks

File:Anatomy and physiology of animals cadriac muscle fibres.jpg *Source*: http://en.wikibooks.org/w/index.php?title=File:Anatomy_and_physiology_of_animals_cadriac_muscle_fibres.jpg *License*: Creative Commons Attribution 2.5 *Contributors*: Original uploader was Sunshineconnelly at en.wikibooks

File:Anatomy and physiology of animals motor neuron.jpg *Source*: http://en.wikibooks.org/w/index.php?title=File:Anatomy_and_physiology_of_animals_motor_neuron.jpg *License*: Creative Commons Attribution 2.5 *Contributors*: Original uploader was Sunshineconnelly at en.wikibooks

File:Anatomy and physiology of animals body cavities.jpg *Source*: http://en.wikibooks.org/w/index.php?title=File:Anatomy_and_physiology_of_animals_body_cavities.jpg *License*: Creative Commons Attribution 2.5 *Contributors*: Original uploader was Sunshineconnelly at en.wikibooks

File:Anatomy and physiology of animals forming digestive systems.jpg *Source*: http://en.wikibooks.org/w/index.php?title=File:Anatomy_and_physiology_of_animals_forming_digestive_systems.jpg *License*: Creative Commons Attribution 2.5 *Contributors*: Original uploader was Sunshineconnelly at en.wikibooks

Image:Anatomy and physiology of animals main organs vertebrate body.jpg *Source*: http://en.wikibooks.org/w/index.php?title=File:Anatomy_and_physiology_of_animals_main_organs_vertebrate_body.jpg *License*: Creative Commons Attribution 2.5 *Contributors*: Original uploader was Sunshineconnelly at en.wikibooks. Later version(s) were uploaded by Adrignola at en.wikibooks.

File:Direcoes anatomicas.svg *Source*: http://en.wikibooks.org/w/index.php?title=File:Direcoes_anatomicas.svg *License*: Public Domain *Contributors*: Rhcastilhos

File:TS mouse.JPG *Source*: http://en.wikibooks.org/w/index.php?title=File:TS_mouse.JPG *License*: Creative Commons Attribution-Sharealike 3.0,2.5,2.0,1.0 *Contributors*: Original uploader was Rlawson at en.wikibooks

File:Anatomy and Physiology of Animals - 05 Skin.jpg *Source*: http://en.wikibooks.org/w/index.php?title=File:Anatomy_and_Physiology_of_Animals_-_05_Skin.jpg *License*: Creative Commons Attribution 3.0 *Contributors*: Original uploader was Sunshineconnelly at en.wikibooks

Image:Anatomy and physiology of animals Cross section skin.jpg *Source*: http://en.wikibooks.org/w/index.php?title=File:Anatomy_and_physiology_of_animals_Cross_section_skin.jpg *License*: Creative Commons Attribution 3.0 *Contributors*: Original uploader was Sunshineconnelly at en.wikibooks

Image:Anatomy and physiology of animals Carnivors claw.jpg *Source*: http://en.wikibooks.org/w/index.php?title=File:Anatomy_and_physiology_of_animals_Carnivors_claw.jpg *License*: Creative Commons Attribution 3.0 *Contributors*: Original uploader was Sunshineconnelly at en.wikibooks

Image:Anatomy and physiology of animal Horses hoof.jpg *Source*: http://en.wikibooks.org/w/index.php?title=File:Anatomy_and_physiology_of_animal_Horses_hoof.jpg *License*: Creative Commons Attribution 3.0 *Contributors*: Original uploader was Sunshineconnelly at en.wikibooks

Image:Anatomy and physiology of animals A horn.jpg *Source*: http://en.wikibooks.org/w/index.php?title=File:Anatomy_and_physiology_of_animals_A_horn.jpg *License*: Creative Commons Attribution 3.0 *Contributors*: Original uploader was Sunshineconnelly at en.wikibooks

Image:Anatomy and physiology of animals Deer antler.jpg *Source*: http://en.wikibooks.org/w/index.php?title=File:Anatomy_and_physiology_of_animals_Deer_antler.jpg *License*: Creative Commons Attribution 3.0 *Contributors*: Original uploader was Sunshineconnelly at en.wikibooks

Image:Anatomy and physiology of animals A hair.jpg *Source*: http://en.wikibooks.org/w/index.php?title=File:Anatomy_and_physiology_of_animals_A_hair.jpg *License*: Creative Commons Attribution 3.0 *Contributors*: Original uploader was Sunshineconnelly at en.wikibooks

Image:Anatomy and physiology of animals Contour feather.jpg *Source*: http://en.wikibooks.org/w/index.php?title=File:Anatomy_and_physiology_of_animals_Contour_feather.jpg *License*: Creative Commons Attribution 3.0 *Contributors*: Original uploader was Sunshineconnelly at en.wikibooks

Image:Anatomy and physiology of animals Down feather.jpg *Source*: http://en.wikibooks.org/w/index.php?title=File:Anatomy_and_physiology_of_animals_Down_feather.jpg *License*: Creative Commons Attribution 3.0 *Contributors*: Original uploader was Sunshineconnelly at en.wikibooks

Image:Anatomy and physiology of animals Pin feather.jpg *Source*: http://en.wikibooks.org/w/index.php?title=File:Anatomy_and_physiology_of_animals_Pin_feather.jpg *License*: Creative Commons Attribution 3.0 *Contributors*: Original uploader was Sunshineconnelly at en.wikibooks

Image:Anatomy and physiology of animals Mammary gland.jpg *Source*: http://en.wikibooks.org/w/index.php?title=File:Anatomy_and_physiology_of_animals_Mammary_gland.jpg *License*: Creative Commons Attribution 3.0 *Contributors*: Original uploader was Sunshineconnelly at en.wikibooks

Image:Anatomy and physiology of animals Hair muscle.jpg *Source*: http://en.wikibooks.org/w/index.php?title=File:Anatomy_and_physiology_of_animals_Hair_muscle.jpg *License*: Creative Commons Attribution 3.0 *Contributors*: Original uploader was Sunshineconnelly at en.wikibooks

Image:Anatomy and physiology of animals Reduction of heat loss by skin.jpg *Source*: http://en.wikibooks.org/w/index.php?title=File:Anatomy_and_physiology_of_animals_Reduction_of_heat_loss_by_skin.jpg *License*: Creative Commons Attribution 3.0 *Contributors*: Original uploader was Sunshineconnelly at en.wikibooks

Image:Anatomy and physiology of animals Increase heat loss by skin.jpg *Source*: http://en.wikibooks.org/w/index.php?title=File:Anatomy_and_physiology_of_animals_Increase_heat_loss_by_skin.jpg *License*: Creative Commons Attribution 3.0 *Contributors*: Original uploader was Sunshineconnelly at en.wikibooks

File:Anatomy and Physiology of Animals - 06 Skeleton.jpg *Source*: http://en.wikibooks.org/w/index.php?title=File:Anatomy_and_Physiology_of_Animals_-_06_Skeleton.jpg *License*: Creative Commons Attribution 3.0 *Contributors*: Original uploader was Sunshineconnelly at en.wikibooks

Image:Anatomy and physiology of animals Mamalian skeleton.jpg *Source*: http://en.wikibooks.org/w/index.php?title=File:Anatomy_and_physiology_of_animals_Mamalian_skeleton.jpg *License*: Creative Commons Attribution 3.0 *Contributors*: Original uploader was Sunshineconnelly at en.wikibooks

Image:Vertebra.JPG *Source*: http://en.wikibooks.org/w/index.php?title=File:Vertebra.JPG *License*: Creative Commons Attribution-Sharealike 3.0,2.5,2.0,1.0 *Contributors*: Original uploader was Rlawson at en.wikibooks

Image:Anatomy and physiology of animals Regions of a vertebral column.jpg *Source*: http://en.wikibooks.org/w/index.php?title=File:Anatomy_and_physiology_of_animals_Regions_of_a_vertebral_column.jpg *License*: Creative Commons Attribution 3.0 *Contributors*: Original uploader was Sunshineconnelly at en.wikibooks

Image:Anatomy and physiology of animals Dogs skull.jpg *Source*: http://en.wikibooks.org/w/index.php?title=File:Anatomy_and_physiology_of_animals_Dogs_skull.jpg *License*: Creative Commons Attribution 3.0 *Contributors*: Original uploader was Sunshineconnelly at en.wikibooks

Image:Anatomy and physiology of animals Ribs.jpg *Source*: http://en.wikibooks.org/w/index.php?title=File:Anatomy_and_physiology_of_animals_Ribs.jpg *License*: Creative Commons Attribution 3.0 *Contributors*: Original uploader was Sunshineconnelly at en.wikibooks

Image:Forelimb dog corrected.JPG *Source*: http://en.wikibooks.org/w/index.php?title=File:Forelimb_dog_corrected.JPG *License*: Creative Commons Attribution-Sharealike 3.0,2.5,2.0,1.0 *Contributors*: Original uploader was Rlawson at en.wikibooks

Image:Hind limb dog corrected.JPG *Source*: http://en.wikibooks.org/w/index.php?title=File:Hind_limb_dog_corrected.JPG *License*: Creative Commons Attribution-Sharealike 3.0,2.5,2.0,1.0 *Contributors*: Original uploader was Rlawson at en.wikibooks

Image:Anatomy and physiology of animals Various vertebrate limbs.jpg *Source*: http://en.wikibooks.org/w/index.php?title=File:Anatomy_and_physiology_of_animals_Various_vertebrate_limbs.jpg *License*: Creative Commons Attribution 3.0 *Contributors*: Original uploader was Sunshineconnelly at en.wikibooks

Image:Anatomy and physiology of animals Forelimb of a horse.jpg *Source*: http://en.wikibooks.org/w/index.php?title=File:Anatomy_and_physiology_of_animals_Forelimb_of_a_horse.jpg *License*: Creative Commons Attribution 3.0 *Contributors*: Original uploader was Sunshineconnelly at en.wikibooks

Image:Anatomy and physiology of animals Valves in a vein.jpg *Source*: http://en.wikibooks.org/w/index.php?title=File:Anatomy_and_physiology_of_animals_Valves_in_a_vein.jpg *License*: Creative Commons Attribution 3.0 *Contributors*: Original uploader was Sunshineconnelly at en.wikibooks

Image:Anatomy and physiology of animals Main arteries and veins of the horse.jpg *Source*: http://en.wikibooks.org/w/index.php?title=File:Anatomy_and_physiology_of_animals_Main_arteries_and_veins_of_the_horse.jpg *License*: Creative Commons Attribution 3.0 *Contributors*: Original uploadeCC-BY-3.0.

Image:Main arteries of the body.jpg *Source*: http://en.wikibooks.org/w/index.php?title=File:Main_arteries_of_the_body.jpg *License*: Creative Commons Attribution 3.0 *Contributors*: Original uploader was Sunshineconnelly at en.wikibooks

File:Anatomy and Physiology of Animals - 09 Respiratory.jpg *Source*: http://en.wikibooks.org/w/index.php?title=File:Anatomy_and_Physiology_of_Animals_-_09_Respiratory.jpg *License*: Creative Commons Attribution 3.0 *Contributors*: Original uploader was Sunshineconnelly at en.wikibooks

File:Anatomy and physiology of animals Alveoli with blood supply.jpg *Source*: http://en.wikibooks.org/w/index.php?title=File:Anatomy_and_physiology_of_animals_Alveoli_with_blood_supply.jpg *License*: Creative Commons Attribution 3.0 *Contributors*: Original uploader was Sunshineconnelly at en.wikibooks. Later version(s) were uploaded by Adrignola, Rlawson at en.wikibooks.

File:Anatomy and physiology of animals cs of an alveolus.jpg *Source*: http://en.wikibooks.org/w/index.php?title=File:Anatomy_and_physiology_of_animals_cs_of_an_alveolus.jpg *License*: Creative Commons Attribution 3.0 *Contributors*: Original uploader was Sunshineconnelly at en.wikibooks. Later version(s) were uploaded by Adrignola at en.wikibooks.

File:The respiratory system.jpg *Source*: http://en.wikibooks.org/w/index.php?title=File:The_respiratory_system.jpg *License*: Creative Commons Attribution 3.0 *Contributors*: Original uploader was Sunshineconnelly at en.wikibooks

Image:Anatomy and physiology of animals Inspiration & expiration.jpg *Source*: http://en.wikibooks.org/w/index.php?title=File:Anatomy_and_physiology_of_animals_Inspiration_&_expiration.jpg *License*: Creative Commons Attribution 3.0 *Contributors*: Original uploader was Sunshineconnelly at en.wikibooks. Later version(s) were uploaded by Adrignola at en.wikibooks.

Image:Anatomy and physiology of animals Lung volumes.jpg *Source*: http://en.wikibooks.org/w/index.php?title=File:Anatomy_and_physiology_of_animals_Lung_volumes.jpg *License*: Creative Commons Attribution 3.0 *Contributors*: Original uploader was Sunshineconnelly at en.wikibooks. Later version(s) were uploaded by Adrignola at en.wikibooks.

File:Anatomy and Physiology of Animals - 10 Lymphatic.jpg *Source*: http://en.wikibooks.org/w/index.php?title=File:Anatomy_and_Physiology_of_Animals_-_10_Lymphatic.jpg *License*: Creative Commons Attribution 3.0 *Contributors*: Original uploader was Sunshineconnelly at en.wikibooks

Image:Anatomy and physiology of animals Capillary bed with lymphatic capilaries.jpg *Source*: http://en.wikibooks.org/w/index.php?title=File:Anatomy_and_physiology_of_animals_Capillary_bed_with_lymphatic_capilaries.jpg *License*: Creative Commons Attribution 3.0 *Contributors*: Original uploader was Sunshineconnelly at en.wikibooks

Image:Anatomy and physiology of animals Lymphatic system.jpg *Source*: http://en.wikibooks.org/w/index.php?title=File:Anatomy_and_physiology_of_animals_Lymphatic_system.jpg *License*: Creative Commons Attribution 3.0 *Contributors*: Original uploader was Sunshineconnelly at en.wikibooks

Image:Anatomy and physiology of animals Circulation of lymph w major lymph nodes.jpg *Source*: http://en.wikibooks.org/w/index.php?title=File:Anatomy_and_physiology_of_animals_Circulation_of_lymph_w_major_lymph_nodes.jpg *License*: Creative Commons Attribution 3.0 *Contributors*: Original uploader was Sunshineconnelly at en.wikibooks

Image:Anatomy and physiology of animals Lymph node.jpg *Source*: http://en.wikibooks.org/w/index.php?title=File:Anatomy_and_physiology_of_animals_Lymph_node.jpg *License*: Creative Commons Attribution 3.0 *Contributors*: Original uploader was Sunshineconnelly at en.wikibooks

File:Anatomy and Physiology of Animals - 11 Digestion.jpg *Source*: http://en.wikibooks.org/w/index.php?title=File:Anatomy_and_Physiology_of_Animals_-_11_Digestion.jpg *License*: Creative Commons Attribution 3.0 *Contributors*: Original uploader was Sunshineconnelly at en.wikibooks

Image:Anatomy and physiology of animals From ingestion to egestion.jpg *Source*: http://en.wikibooks.org/w/index.php?title=File:Anatomy_and_physiology_of_animals_From_ingestion_to_egestion.jpg *License*: Creative Commons Attribution 3.0 *Contributors*: Original uploader was Sunshineconnelly at en.wikibooks

Image:Anatomy and physiology of animals Typical mammalian gut.jpg *Source*: http://en.wikibooks.org/w/index.php?title=File:Anatomy_and_physiology_of_animals_Typical_mammalian_gut.jpg *License*: Creative Commons Attribution 3.0 *Contributors*: Original uploader was Sunshineconnelly at en.wikibooks

Image:Anatomy and physiology of animals Salivary glands.jpg *Source*: http://en.wikibooks.org/w/index.php?title=File:Anatomy_and_physiology_of_animals_Salivary_glands.jpg *License*: Creative Commons Attribution 3.0 *Contributors*: Original uploader was Sunshineconnelly at en.wikibooks

Image:Anatomy and physiology of animals Section through head of a dog.jpg *Source*: http://en.wikibooks.org/w/index.php?title=File:Anatomy_and_physiology_of_animals_Section_through_head_of_a_dog.jpg *License*: Creative Commons Attribution 3.0 *Contributors*: Original uploader was Sunshineconnelly at en.wikibooks

Image:Anatomy and physiology of animals Stucture of tooth.jpg *Source*: http://en.wikibooks.org/w/index.php?title=File:Anatomy_and_physiology_of_animals_Stucture_of_tooth.jpg *License*: Creative Commons Attribution 3.0 *Contributors*: Original uploader was Sunshineconnelly at en.wikibooks

Image:Anatomy and physiology of animals Sheeps skull.jpg *Source*: http://en.wikibooks.org/w/index.php?title=File:Anatomy_and_physiology_of_animals_Sheeps_skull.jpg *License*: Creative Commons Attribution 3.0 *Contributors*: Original uploader was Sunshineconnelly at en.wikibooks

Image:Anatomy and physiology of animals Peristalis.jpg *Source*: http://en.wikibooks.org/w/index.php?title=File:Anatomy_and_physiology_of_animals_Peristalis.jpg *License*: Creative Commons Attribution 3.0 *Contributors*: Original uploader was Sunshineconnelly at en.wikibooks

Image:Anatomy and physiology of animals Stomach.jpg *Source*: http://en.wikibooks.org/w/index.php?title=File:Anatomy_and_physiology_of_animals_Stomach.jpg *License*: Creative Commons Attribution 3.0 *Contributors*: Original uploader was Sunshineconnelly at en.wikibooks

Image:Anatomy and physiology of animals Wall of small intestine showing villi.jpg *Source*: http://en.wikibooks.org/w/index.php?title=File:Anatomy_and_physiology_of_animals_Wall_of_small_intestine_showing_villi.jpg *License*: Creative Commons Attribution 3.0 *Contributors*: Original uploader was Sunshineconnelly at en.wikibooks

Image:Anatomy and physiology of animals The rumen.jpg *Source*: http://en.wikibooks.org/w/index.php?title=File:Anatomy_and_physiology_of_animals_The_rumen.jpg *License*: Creative Commons Attribution 3.0 *Contributors*: Original uploader was Sunshineconnelly at en.wikibooks

Image:Anatomy and physiology of animals Gut of a rabbit.jpg *Source*: http://en.wikibooks.org/w/index.php?title=File:Anatomy_and_physiology_of_animals_Gut_of_a_rabbit.jpg *License*: Creative Commons Attribution 3.0 *Contributors*: Original uploader was Sunshineconnelly at en.wikibooks

Image:Anatomy and physiology of animals Stomach & small intestine of hen.jpg *Source*: http://en.wikibooks.org/w/index.php?title=File:Anatomy_and_physiology_of_animals_Stomach_&_small_intestine_of_hen.jpg *License*: Creative Commons Attribution 3.0 *Contributors*: Original uploader was Sunshineconnelly at en.wikibooks

Image:Anatomy and physiology of animals Liver, gall bladder & pancreas.jpg *Source*: http://en.wikibooks.org/w/index.php?title=File:Anatomy_and_physiology_of_animals_Liver,_gall_bladder_&_pancreas.jpg *License*: Creative Commons Attribution 3.0 *Contributors*: Original uploader was Sunshineconnelly at en.wikibooks

Image:Anatomy and physiology of animals Control of glucose by the liver.jpg *Source*: http://en.wikibooks.org/w/index.php?title=File:Anatomy_and_physiology_of_animals_Control_of_glucose_by_the_liver.jpg *License*: Creative Commons Attribution 3.0 *Contributors*: Original uploader was Sunshineconnelly at en.wikibooks

Image:Anatomy and physiology of animals Summary of the main functions of the different regions of the gut.jpg *Source*: http://en.wikibooks.org/w/index.php?title=File:Anatomy_and_physiology_of_animals_Summary_of_the_main_functions_of_the_different_regions_of_the_gut.jpg *License*: Creative Commons Attribution 3.0 *Contributors*: Original uploader was Sunshineconnelly at en.wikibooks

File:Anatomy and Physiology of Animals - 12 Urinary.jpg *Source*: http://en.wikibooks.org/w/index.php?title=File:Anatomy_and_Physiology_of_Animals_-_12_Urinary.jpg *License*: Creative Commons Attribution 3.0 *Contributors*: Original uploader was Sunshineconnelly at en.wikibooks

Image:Anatomy and physiology of animals Water in the body.jpg *Source*: http://en.wikibooks.org/w/index.php?title=File:Anatomy_and_physiology_of_animals_Water_in_the_body.jpg *License*: Creative Commons Attribution 3.0 *Contributors*: Original uploader was Sunshineconnelly at en.wikibooks

Image:Urinary_System_of_Dog.JPG *Source*: http://en.wikibooks.org/w/index.php?title=File:Urinary_System_of_Dog.JPG *License*: Creative Commons Attribution 3.0 *Contributors*: Original uploader was Sunshineconnelly at en.wikibooks

Image:Anatomy and physiology of animals Urinary system.jpg *Source*: http://en.wikibooks.org/w/index.php?title=File:Anatomy_and_physiology_of_animals_Urinary_system.jpg *License*: Creative Commons Attribution 3.0 *Contributors*: Original uploader was Sunshineconnelly at en.wikibooks. Later version(s) were uploaded by Rlawson at en.wikibooks.

License

Printed in Great Britain
by Amazon.co.uk, Ltd.,
Marston Gate.